THE PREPPER'S ULTIMATE FIRST AID BIBLE

PROVIDE MEDICAL CARE WHEN SOCIETY COLLAPSE

by
Robert Freeman

© Copyright 2023 by Robert Freeman - All rights reserved.

This document is geared towards providing exact and reliable information in regard to the topic and issue covered. The publication is sold with the idea that the publisher is not required to render accounting, officially permitted, or otherwise, qualified services. If advice is necessary, legal, or professional, a practiced individual in the profession should be ordered.

From a Declaration of Principles, which was accepted and approved equally by a Committee of the American Bar Association and a Committee of Publishers and Associations. In no way is it legal to reproduce, duplicate, or transmit any part of this document in either electronic means or in printed format. Recording of this publication is strictly prohibited, and any storage of this document is not allowed unless with written permission from the publisher. All rights reserved.

The information provided herein is stated to be truthful and consistent, in that any liability, in terms of inattention or otherwise, by any usage or abuse of any policies, processes, or directions contained within is the solitary and utter responsibility of the recipient reader. Under no circumstances will any legal responsibility or blame be held against the publisher for any reparation, damages, or monetary loss due to the information herein, either directly or indirectly. Respective authors own all copyrights not held by the publisher. The information herein is offered for informational purposes solely and is universal as so. The presentation of the information is without contract or any type of guarantee assurance. The trademarks that are used are without any consent, and the publication of the trademark is without permission or backing by the trademark owner. All trademarks and brands within this book are for clarifying purposes only and are owned by the owners themselves, not affiliated with this document.

TABLE OF CONTENTS

Chapter 1: INTRODUCTION TO FIRST AID 6

REASONS WHY BASIC FIRST AID KNOWLEDGE IS IMPORTANT 18

SURVIVAL FIRST AID 21

Chapter 2: HOW TO PERFORM A FIRST AID ASSESSMENT 33

THE RECOVERY POSITION IN FIRST AID 35

Chapter 3: CPR GUIDE 44

Chapter 4: BITES AND STINGS 51

Chapter 5: CHOKING 59

Chapter 6: BURNS 62

Chapter 7: SPRAINS AND STRAINS 68

Chapter 8: DISLOCATIONS 72

Chapter 9: HEAD INJURY 78

Chapter 10: POISONING 85

Chapter 11: FROSTBITE 93

Chapter 12: BURNS AND SCALDS 96

Chapter 13: HEART ATTACK 99

Chapter 14: DIABETES 103

Chapter 15: ASTHMA 107

Chapter 16: BLEEDING 112

Chapter 17: STROKE 116

Chapter 18: EPILEPSY SEIZURES 120

Chapter 19: HYPOTHERMIA 124

Chapter 20: TICK BITE 133

Chapter 21: SHOCK 137

Chapter 22: PANIC ATTACK 142

Chapter 23: BREATHING DIFFICULTIES 152

HOW TO TAKE A PULSE IN FIRST AID 159

Chapter 24: RESPIRATORY RATE FOR ADULTS AND CHILDREN..161

Chapter 25: THE ULTIMATE PREPPER FIRST AID KIT..170

CONCLUSION..182

BONUS #1..184

BONUS #2..185

BONUS #3..186

BONUSES

ON THE LAST PAGES OF THIS GUIDE YOU WILL FIND THE WAY TO GET THESE 3 FANTASTIC BONUSES FOR FREE:

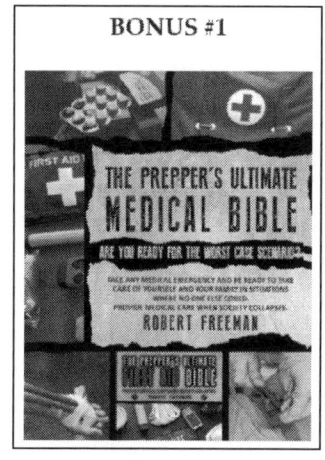

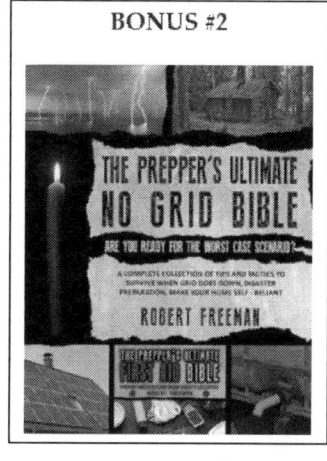

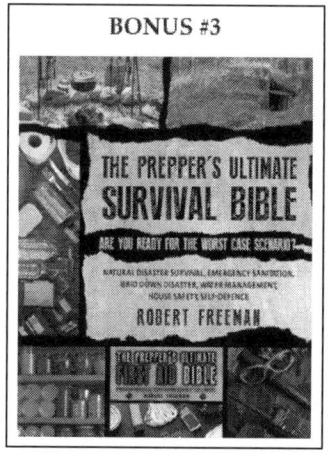

Topics:

SURVIVAL MEDICINE

MEDICAL SUPPLIES

HYGIENE AND SANITATIOn

THE MASS CASUALTY INCIDENT

DENTAL CARE

INFECTIONS

ALLERGIC EMERGENCIES

INJURIES

Topics:

CAUSES OF A GRID DOWN

OFF GRID POWER SOURCES

SELF-RELIANT HOME

FOOD SHORTAGE

WATER MANAGEMENT

NO-GRID SECURITY

COMPOST WATER HEATER

SOLAR BATTERY CHARGER

Topics:

EMERGENCY PREPAREDNESS

BUG OUT

BUG-IN

PREPPER FOOD

WATER SURVIVAL GUIDE

BECOME A PREPPER

FOODS TO STOCKPILE

PREPAREDNESS CHECKLIST

Chapter 1: INTRODUCTION TO FIRST AID

You might get injured or ill at any time, or someone close to you could. You might be able to prevent a minor injury from turning worse by using basic first aid. In an extreme medical situation, you could even be able to save a life.

This is why learning the fundamentals of first aid is so crucial. You could consider enrolling in a first aid course to expand on the knowledge you get from this.

Definition of First Aid

First aid refers to the basic medical care given to someone suddenly unwell or injured.

First aid can also refer to the initial care given to a patient during a medical emergency. They might be able to survive with this support until help from professionals arrives.

In other situations, first aid is limited to the treatment given to a small-wound victim. For instance, small burns, wounds, and insect stings can frequently be treated with first aid alone.

Steps for Emergency Situations

Adhere to these three fundamental steps in the event of an emergency:

1. Scan the area for any signs of danger.

Watch for anything harmful, such as violent individuals, falling objects, or fire signs. If you feel your safety is at risk, get out of the situation and call for help.

Examine the wounded or ill person's condition when the scene is safe. Move them only if it is necessary to keep them safe.

2. Provide care

Stay with the ill or wounded individual until proficient aid arrives if it is safe for you to do so. Try to keep them quiet, comfort them, and cover them with a warm blanket. If you are proficient in basic first aid, try to treat any potentially fatal wounds they may have.

If you believe your safety is in jeopardy at any moment throughout the incident, take steps to remove yourself from danger.

First Aid Bandage

Adhesive bandages are frequently useful for covering small burns, scratches, and wounds. Larger wounds may need to be covered and protected with a roller bandage or a clean gauze pad.

Use these procedures to apply a roller bandage to a wound:

Keep the wounded area still.

Cover the wound gently but firmly wrap the bandage over the injured limb or body part.

Use safety pins or adhesive tape to secure the bandage.

The bandage should be applied tightly enough to hold it in place without obstructing blood flow.

To examine the circulation in a bandaged limb, pinch one of the person's toenails or fingernails until the color disappears. After releasing, go for two seconds. If color doesn't return, the bandage is too tight and has to be adjusted.

First Aid for Burns

Pay attention for any burns that:

- span a substantial portion of skin;
- are found on the buttocks, hands, face, groin, or feet of the individual;
- been brought on by coming into contact with electricity or chemicals.

Those are very difficult to manage so in the treatment be careful not to cause further damage.

To treat a mild burn, apply cold water to the burned area for up to fifteen minutes. If that isn't feasible, treat the region with a cold compress. Don't put ice on burnt tissue. It can cause more harm.

Over-the-counter pain killers can aid with pain relief. For small burns, lidocaine, aloe vera gel, or lotion can also help ease discomfort.

Apply an antibiotic ointment and wrap the burn loosely with clean gauze to help prevent infection. Find out when it's appropriate to schedule follow-up treatment with a doctor.

First Aid CPR

You could intervene if you witness someone pass out or discover someone unconscious. Approach the unconscious individual and start CPR if the environment surrounding them is safe.

You can do hands-only CPR to help someone stay alive until expert aid arrives, even if you have never had official training in the procedure.

How to treat an adult with hands-only CPR:

With one hand on top of the other, place both hands on the middle of the chest.

At around 100 to 120 compressions per minute, press straight down to continually press their chest.

You may count at the proper pace by compressing your chest to the tune of "Crazy in Love" by Beyoncé or "Staying Alive" by the Bee Gees.

Hold off on chest compressions until assistance from a medical expert comes.

Discover how to do CPR on a baby or toddler and how to perform rescue breathing in addition to chest compressions.

First Aid for Bee Sting

A bee sting might be a medical emergency for certain people. If someone is experiencing an allergic response to a bee sting assist them in finding and using any epinephrine auto-injectors they may have, such as an EpiPen. As help arrives, urge them to maintain their composure.

Most of the time, a bee sting victim who is not exhibiting any symptoms of an allergic response can be treated independently without medical assistance.

If the stinger is still embedded under the skin, gently scrape a credit card or other flat item across the skin to remove the stinger. Next, to lessen discomfort and swelling, wash the affected region with soap and water and use a cold compress for up to ten minutes at a time.

Consider using calamine lotion or a paste made of baking soda and water to the affected region several times a day to relieve any itching or pain caused by the sting.

First Aid for Bleeding Noses

When treating a nosebleed patient, instruct them to:

Take a seat and lean their head forward.

Seal the nose shut by applying pressure with the thumb and index finger.

Keep applying this pressure nonstop for five minutes.

Examine again, and repeat until the bleeding stops.

You can pinch or force their nose shut if you have vinyl or nitrile gloves.

Get immediate medical attention if the bleeding persists for more than twenty minutes. If an injury results in a nosebleed, the patient should also have follow-up care.

First Aid for Heatstroke

Heat exhaustion can arise from your body overheating. Heat exhaustion may lead to heatstroke if left untreated. This is a medical emergency with possible life-threatening consequences.

Encourage someone hot to take a nap in a cool place. Take off extra layers of clothes and try the following methods to help them cool down:

Put a cold, wet sheet over them.

Place a damp, cold cloth over the back of their neck.

Use cold water to sponge them.

If they exhibit any of the following heatstroke signs or symptoms, it means that it is very serious:

- vomiting or nausea
- mental disarray
- a fever of 40°C (104°F) or higher
- seizures
- fainting

If they aren't unconscious or vomiting, encourage them to take a sports drink or sip cool water.

Heart Attack First Aid

If you believe someone is having a heart attack assist them in finding and taking nitroglycerin if it has been prescribed. Calm them and cover them with a blanket till aid from a professional source arrives.

Remove any tight clothing around their neck and chest if they are having trouble breathing. If they pass out, do CPR.

First Aid Kit for Babies

It's a good idea to carry a fully packed first aid kit in your car and house as a precaution against future crises. You may construct your first aid kits or purchase preassembled ones.

If you have a baby, you may need to add infant-appropriate items to your basic first aid kit or replace some items. For instance, a baby thermometer and acetaminophen or ibuprofen should be in your pack.

Additionally, it's essential to keep the kit out of your baby's reach.

First Aid Kit List

You never know when you might need to do basic first aid. One way to be ready for anything is to keep a fully supplied first aid kit in your car and your house. Keeping a first aid kit at work is also a smart idea.

Many first aid groups, pharmacies, and outdoor recreation retailers sell preassembled first aid kits. Alternatively, you can use items from a drugstore to make your first aid pack.

Standard first aid supplies ought to contain the following:

- varied-sized adhesive bandages
- roller bandages with different sizes
- absorbent compress dressings
- adhesive cloth tape
- triangle-shaped bandages
- sterile gauze pads
- aspirin
- ibuprofen or acetaminophen
- antiseptic wipes
- hydrocortisone cream
- antibiotic ointment
- blanket
- calamine lotion
- safety pins
- nitrile or vinyl gloves
- instant cold pack
- scissors
- thermometer
- tweezers
- breathing barrier
- first aid manual

It's a good idea to include a list of your doctors, emergency contact information, and prescription drugs in your first aid kits.

Outlook

When administering first aid, keeping oneself safe from infectious diseases and other dangers is critical.

To better defend oneself:

- always be sure there are no dangers to your safety before approaching an ill or injured individual;
- keep your hands away from blood, vomit, and other body fluids;
- while treating someone who has an open wound or while doing rescue breathing, put on protective gear like vinyl or nitrile gloves or a breathing barrier;
- after administering first aid, quickly wash your hands with soap and water;
- sometimes, simple first aid can prevent a small issue from worsening.

First aid in a medical emergency might potentially save a life. Someone should get follow-up treatment from a medical expert if they have a significant sickness or injury.

What Is a Splint?

A splint is a piece of medical equipment intended to immobilize and shield an injured body part from further harm.

When someone breaks a bone, splinting is frequently performed to stabilize the injury until they can be sent to the hospital for more intensive care. If you have a significant sprain or strain in one of your limbs, you can also utilize it.

When positioned correctly, a hard splint can reduce discomfort by preventing movement of the injured region.

If you or a loved one sustains an injury at home or while engaging in an activity like hiking, you can make a temporary splint of items lying around.

The Supplies Needed to Splint an Injury

You'll need something stiff to stabilize the fracture as soon as you create a splint. Among the things you can utilize are:

- a newspaper wrapped up and a thick stick
- a plank or board
- a wrapped-up towel

When handling objects like sticks or boards with sharp edges that might splinter, cushion them thoroughly by wrapping them in fabric. Additional strain on the injury can also be lessened with proper cushioning.

Additionally, you'll need something to secure the improvised splint in position. It will work with shoelaces, belts, ropes, and strips of cloth. If you have medical tape, you can use that as well.

Avoid putting commercial tape, like duct tape, up against someone's skin.

Applying a Splint

The steps listed below will teach you how to put on a splint.

1. Take care of any bleeding

If there is any bleeding, take care of it before applying the splint. Applying pressure directly to the wound will effectively halt the bleeding.

2. Use cushioning

Next, affix a bandage, a gauze square, or a piece of fabric.

The bodily part that has to be splinted should not be moved. You risk inadvertently doing additional harm while attempting to straighten a fractured bone or malformed bodily component.

3. Position the splint.

Position the handmade splint carefully to cover the joint above and below the damage.

For instance, position the stiff support item beneath the forearm if you are splinting it. Next, fasten it to the arm by taping or tying it immediately above the elbow and below the wrist.

Keep your ties away from the region that is hurt. Splints should be fastened securely enough to keep the affected body part immobile but not so securely that the wearer's circulation is interrupted by the ties.

4. Be alert for any indications of shock or impaired blood flow.

After the splinting, you should periodically inspect the surrounding regions for evidence of reduced blood flow.

Loosen the knots holding the splint if the limbs look pale, bloated, or blue-tinged.

The splint might be too tight due to swelling after the event. In addition to feeling tightness, check for a pulse. In case it's weak, unfasten the knots.

Try to release the knots if the wounded individual complains that the splint hurts. Next, make sure no ties are applied directly over any wounds.

You should take the splint off if these remedies don't work and the patient is still experiencing pain from it.

The injured individual may be in shock, manifesting as short, fast breathing, or dizzy. Try to lay them down in this situation to not stress the wounded body part. You want to get their head below heart level and raise their legs.

5. Get medical attention

Once the damaged body part cannot move following the splint's application, if available in the scenario you are in, look for a dressing station with trained staff.

They will require further care in addition to a checkup.

Splinting the Hand

It is particularly challenging to paralyze the hand. Here are a few pointers for creating a homemade hand splint.

1. Stop any bleeding

Take care of any exposed wounds and stop any bleeding first.

2. Put something in your hand's palm.

Next, put a wad of cloth in the wounded person's hand's palm. You can use a tennis ball, a ball of socks, or a washcloth.

Have them gently round the thing with their fingertips.

3. Use padding

After the person's fingers are closed around the object, loosely place padding between their fingers.

Next, cover the entire hand—from the fingers to the wrist—with a big piece of gauze or fabric. The material should stretch from the thumb to the pinkie on the hand.

4. Tighten the padding.

Lastly, fasten the material firmly with ties or tape. Don't forget to keep the fingertips exposed. You can then look for indications of impaired circulation.

When to Get in Touch With a Doctor

Is difficult to find in a TEOTWAWKI scenario but if possible, look for a dressing place for the following cases::

- bone that is visible through the skin
- an open wound where the injury occurred
- pulse loss at the site of injury
- lack of feeling in the wounded limb's fingers or toes that have become numb and bluish
- a sensation of warmth surrounding the wound

Setting up appropriate medical care for the wounded individual should be your priority when dealing with an emergency incident.

While waiting for qualified help or to assist with transportation, a homemade splint can be effective first aid.

To ensure that your splinting doesn't exacerbate the injury, you must closely adhere to the guidelines.

REASONS WHY BASIC FIRST AID KNOWLEDGE IS IMPORTANT

Gaining First Aid knowledge provides advantages. There is no assurance that individuals won't experience bodily harm, disease, or trauma, and accidents are unavoidable. The finest thing people can do in an accident, tragedy, or other catastrophe is to be ready.

Many factors prevent people from receiving the training and education needed to properly administer first aid.

- Fear of making a mistake
- False beliefs about the price of training
- Lack of sufficient time
- Not sure where to obtain instruction

A skilled individual has the power to save lives and change the world. In contrast, an untrained individual is probably perplexed and unsure of what to do in an emergency.

It just takes a few hours to finish a first aid course, but the information gained will give a person the tools they need to handle any situation.

One acquires knowledge in First Aid through training. These are the top 4 reasons that first aid instruction is crucial.

First Aid Save Lives

Millions of individuals suffer injuries each year that result in death or serious injury due to poor reaction times or delayed help. The willingness of the bystander to assist makes a significant difference between those who survive and those who do not. When patients get basic life support while an ambulance is being dispatched, their chances of survival are doubled.

First Aid Reduces Pain

Since pain can alter respiration, heart rate, and blood pressure, providing pain relief is crucial. Before medical emergency services arrive, simple measures like using an ice pack or giving yourself a brief rub will assist in reducing and lessening the pain.

First Aid Builds Self-Assurance

Significant first aid training instills confidence, eliminating or replacing the anxiety of assisting other victims in an emergency. Skilled individuals are eager to intervene and offer immediate assistance to those in need.

First Aid Boosts Security

The protective barrier that keeps the threat at bay can be automated with first aid training. Everybody attending the program gains the ability to properly analyze the situation, respond effectively, and pay more attention to safety in their own home, places of employment, and communities.

First Aid Stops the Crisis from Getting Worse

Having the fundamental understanding necessary to manage difficult circumstances helps prevent things from worsening. Until the emergency response is prepared, the victim's health can be stabilized with prompt and temporary medical attention.

First Aid Raises Living Standards

Those who have received the appropriate training in first aid can live without experiencing more trauma, fear, or danger. One becomes more conscious of their lifestyle choices and behaviors to reduce the chance of developing health and safety issues when well-informed about these topics.

One acquires knowledge in First Aid through training.

We implore everyone to serve one another without letting fear, time, or money stand in the way. There's never been a greater opportunity to pick up new abilities that could save lives than now.

SURVIVAL FIRST AID

Emergencies related to medicine occur often. From little cuts and scratches to broken bones and severe injuries, having the right first aid supplies on hand can greatly help.

This book reviews and recommends the best first aid kits, equipment, and training resources currently in the market. We beg you to have the necessary items in your home, vehicle, place of employment, school, and place of worship so that you are always ready. Additionally, we beg you to pursue professional training so that you can identify and manage diseases well enough to recommend patients to specialists.

Not only can having the right tools help, but knowing how to use them properly can immediately make a bad situation good. Let's go on now!

First Aid Kits

There are many different styles of first aid kits. A quick online search will produce many kits in all sizes and shapes. How are you going to choose one? What products should be housed inside? The options below are the ones we think are best.

Basic First Aid Kits

Basic first aid kits include supplies for treating simple cuts, scratches, and light discomfort. These include bandages, small bandages, analgesics, antiseptics, etc.

Easy kits are perfect to slip into a handbag or coat pocket. They come in little bags with zippers. For instance, they are quite effective in stopping little bleeding.

Standard First Aid Kits

A standard first-aid pack contains several hundred first-aid supplies. Beyond the essentials, the kit contains smaller bandages and pads, antiseptics, adhesives, wraps, and medications. They come in pouches, clam-shell containers, or molle pouches.

These kits are still made for very straightforward situations. The majority of the time, they are quite beneficial.

Comprehensive First Aid Kits

Expanded first aid kits can contain supplies like chest seals, irrigation syringes, pressure bandages, tourniquets, splints, and more. The intended audience is those with a bit more technical training. It is unusual to utilize these materials for social events in the home. Shooting incidents, outdoor trips, and athletic activities may require equipment and training.

Trauma Kit

A trauma kit consists of sophisticated equipment and a supply bundle. Neck restraints, sprints, pressure cuffs, airway attachments, suture kits, and other complex equipment improve this set.

Reusable Supplies

Some first aid kits are made mostly of replenished materials. Each item is given in multiples so that someone can restock an existing first aid kit. To replace finished supplies, they could carry medications, bandages, pads, gauze, etc.

Choosing a First Aid Kit

The kind of first aid bundle you choose should match your level of training. You should use each component in your kit to your pleasure. Knowing what to use and when to apply it correctly is your duty. As first responders will tell you, using first aid supplies improperly could worsen an already dire situation.

Experience: it is recommended that you have first aid kits and supplies appropriate for your level of experience and training.

This is how to choose:

- Location: Consider the surroundings and the resources available to you. Emergency circumstances that occur in a religious setting are probably not the same as ones that would occur in an athletic setting. Keeping emergency supplies on hand is crucial since traveling to a hospital in the great outdoors can be difficult.
- Persons: Whom are you responsible for? To whom is your group addressed? Who else has experience in the medical field?
- Training: What degree of instruction in first aid have you completed? Whichever kit you choose, you need to know how to use each of its parts properly.
- Mobility: Do you always need to carry a first aid kit with you? Should it stay in place or be fastened to the wall?

If you're unsure what to use, get a first aid kit with more supplies than you know how to utilize. Research it online or consult a medical professional for more guidance when the box comes. In most cases, it is better to be more structured.

Levels of First Aid Kits

Each of us has a different background and level of training in emergencies and first aid. It is advised that you obtain as much as you can. You can't predict when you might require it.

The general levels that you could be in are as follows:

First Aid Rookie, Level 0

Basic first aid can be performed by a novice in the field. They might be able to clean a scrape, suggest Asprin for a headache, or apply a Band-Aid to a small cut.

First Level: Boy Scout

We advise everyone to receive Boy Scout-level training. Scouts get training in diagnosing and treating a wide range of typical first-aid accidents and using basic to standard first-aid equipment.

They can usually make a splint or sling for a broken limb or sprained joint, assist someone in breathing again, halt light to moderate bleeding, and more. They can walk through procedures to focus on an issue and provide the necessary assistance. They also possess life-essential abilities.

Level 2-Police/Military

A new level of abilities centered on the traumas encountered in the field is added by military basic training. They are prepared to handle injuries from explosions, gunshot wounds, concussions, and other wartime trauma.

Most non-medical personnel lack the time and expertise to get this degree of first aid training. In all honesty, most circumstances don't call for it.

Level 3: Doctors and EMTs

When it comes to first aid training, medical practitioners are the best. For years, they attended school to learn how to fix the human body. We adore our first responders to emergencies and physicians.

It's unlikely that any of us will ever become proficient first aiders. We will never achieve a college degree, even though we should constantly study.

Select your first aid kit depending on your training

Select a first aid kit based on the degree of training you have. We should all be as ready as Boy Scouts. It should be our knowledge to recognize and handle common diseases and injuries. Acquire first aid equipment to strengthen these abilities.

Suggested First Aid Items

We have developed a suggested survival technique for unexpected survival throughout the years. There are four stages in the system. Personal survival supplies and equipment are the main focus of the first two phases, whereas home or communal supplies and equipment are the main focus of the last two. Each stage's suggested first aid checklist is based on activity, weight, and requirements.

Method of Survival

To be prepared for emergencies, we advise putting up a survival system. The system comes with necessary first aid equipment.

Step 1: Essentials

It is advised that everyone bring the necessities for everyday tasks. Every home and car should be equipped with first aid equipment. At least, we should be able to treat cuts, scrapes, small breaks, etc. Some persons should have more sophisticated materials, including tourniquets and bleed stops.

Step 2: Go-Bags

Go-Bags that have mid-level supplies should be prepared in case of evacuation. We should be somewhat self-sufficient because an evacuation may prevent you from having direct access to a hospital or treatment facility.

You should bring extra stuff with you when you travel outside of civilization. Any wounds or illnesses need to have sufficiently healed for us to return home. We also ought to receive a little further instruction.

Step 3: House Kit (for Family and Home)

The majority of municipalities offer access to medical care. In a SHTF situation this could miss, so you should be able to manage on your own. Some wounds, can require immediate attention as severe bleeding injuries, neck injuries, brain injuries, poisonings, etc. These need rapid first aid. We ought to be prepared.

Stage 4: Large-scale supplies and machinery

We advise storing food, additional toiletries, and equipment (such as a generator) for shelter-at-home scenarios. Effective, long-term first aid is essential if you lack access to critical care.

The Goal of the Staged Approach

Being prepared for emergencies means constantly having the appropriate tools and resources for whatever circumstances arise. You frequently don't have easy access to everyday stuff you could have at home when you're away from home. You may also lack the strength and mass to lift heavy objects.

A staged approach lets you carry the maximum possible without overdoing it.

Improvements to First Aid

Learn how to use a few unique goods to enhance the fundamentals. Include a compression sleeve, tourniquet, pressure bandages, etc.

Instruction in First Aid

Improper use of first aid materials might exacerbate the condition. Infection, increased bleeding, worsening of a break, etc., are all possible.

Get CPR Trained and Certified

Cardiopulmonary resuscitation (CPR) is an emergency procedure that manually preserves intact brain function in a person experiencing cardiac arrest until further steps are taken to restore spontaneous breathing and blood circulation. This is often done in conjunction with artificial ventilation.

Most towns offer options for CPR instruction. Fire departments, medical facilities, clinics, EMTs, etc., frequently provide group training programs. They frequently set aside time to certify people or organizations.

Get Trained in C.E.R.T.

There are C.E.R.T.-certified emergency preparation organizations in many localities. They will meet with groups to teach people how to assist first responders in an emergency. They are eager to offer their information. When a calamity strikes, they hope to increase the number of individuals who can assist.

First Aid Kits and Consistent Instruction

Every home, car, place of business, etc., should have first aid supplies and trained personnel on hand. Emergencies occur frequently. Professionals are trustworthy in important situations, but we should be ready for the possibility that they will be overworked or unavailable at other times.

First Aid Kits for Survival

Having the right equipment at hand can save lives. Identifying your options can be difficult. Most first aid kits are designed to buy you enough time to travel to a hospital so that a medical practitioner can treat your wound or illness.

Here is a list of some of the most popular first-aid equipment and supplies, along with a brief description. You can obtain more details on the raw ingredients and manufacturing procedures by doing a product search.

It is imperative that you receive training in the usage of first aid items. Being equipped with the necessary abilities can be quite helpful in an emergency, regardless of whether you are called upon to do more complex medical procedures or only cure a simple cut or injury.

The sources of these condensed summaries are the manufacturer lists, external websites, and first aid manuals. They are meant to serve as a starting point.

Wipes

1. Alcohol Wipes: A tiny pack of cloth wipes packed with rubbing alcohol that is used to clean a limited area before treatment
2. Sting Relief is a tiny cloth wipe that comes in a tiny pack with sting relief ointment sealed inside to lessen the discomfort caused by insect stings.

Gauze and Dressings

1. Compressed Gauze: A package of gauze is used to clean and treat wounds and injuries; the gauze is compressed within the container to reduce the space in a kit.
2. Gauze pad: A gauze pad covers or treats wounds and injuries. It is often packaged in paper.
3. Gauze roll: A single, generally sealed roll of gauze treats and wraps a wound or injury.
4. Larger gauze or fabric pads used to wrap and treat wounds and injuries are called wound dressings.

Adhesive Bandages

Common: an adhesive bandage for minor cuts, scratches, and abrasions composed of fabric or plastic (the Bandaid brand is popular).

1. Butterfly: a plastic or fabric adhesive bandage used to help seal minor cuts and scratches that resemble stitches
2. Knuckle: a plastic or fabric sticky bandage used to treat minor cuts, scratches, and abrasions on fingers or toes
3. Mole Skin: an adhesive patch of fabric or plastic that lessens friction from shoes on the skin and is meant to prevent and treat blisters.

Medium Bandages

1. Trauma Pad/Dressing: a sizable, solitary pad that is typically wrapped in paper to cover or treat an injury or wound
2. ABD Pads: sterile, very absorbent dressings used for wounds that retain a lot of fluid, frequently stomach injuries.
3. Pressure bandages: A pressure bandage often called an Israeli pressure bandage, is a fabric bandage with a mechanical lever that applies pressure to the wound it has been wrapped.

4. Chest Seals: Designed to stop infection, fluid loss, and air passageway following gunshot or puncture wounds, a chest seal seals a cavity hole.

Elastic Bandages

1. Elastic Roll: a fabric elastic roll (also known as Ace Bandage) used to treat joint injuries; the roll is wrapped around a joint to give it structural support, such as the elbow, knee, etc.
2. Burn dressing: a moist, nonstick pad that is frequently covered in gel to lessen burn effects; it also lessens pain and infection

Pills and Tablets

1. Antacids are little tablets that are swallowed to lessen acid reflux.
2. Tylenol is a little tablet that is swallowed to relieve pain.
3. Asprin: a little tablet administered orally to treat certain blood disorders or lessen pain
4. Ibuprofen is a little tablet that is swallowed to relieve pain.
5. Pepto-Bismol is a little tablet or liquid medication administered orally to relieve upset stomachs or diarrhea.
6. Allergy - Small tablet administered orally to minimize some allergic reactions.
7. Water Purification - small tablet applied directly to water (not taken orally) to purify drinking water
8. Imodium is a little tablet or liquid medication consumed orally to treat upset stomachs or diarrhea.
9. Small oral antibiotic tablets called Bactrim Antibiotics are used to treat urinary tract infections, ear infections, and other conditions.

Liquids, Gels, and Creams

1. A Gel called "antibiotic ointment" is applied to wounds to lessen infection.
2. Disinfectant Spray: spray used on a wound site to lessen infection
3. Burn cream: a lotion applied to a burn site to lessen discomfort and infection
4. Burn Spray: a spray used on a burn site to lessen discomfort and infection
5. To lessen sunburn, apply a cream or gel called sun screen cream to your skin.
6. Use insect repellent, often DEET, on your skin to help you avoid insects.
7. Vaseline: a lubricating and moisturizing gel used to treat and conceal some wounds
8. Water-based liquid saline eye drops cure and cleanse eyes.
9. An antifungal drug called miconazole is used to treat vaginal infections.

Powders

1. Bleed Stop is a powder that crystallizes to clot blood until medical personnel can treat a big wound. Its purpose is to lessen or stop bleeding from wounds.

Ligatures and Splints

1. Triangle Bandage: an arm bandage that forms a sling that hangs around the neck and is used to suspend a fractured or damaged arm
2. An aluminum splint is a strap designed to provide structural support for a toe or finger that has been wounded.
3. Silk tape is an adhesive tape that binds pads and bandages around appendages.
4. Adhesive Roll: adhesive tape is used to encircle appendages with pads and bandages
5. Coban Roles are flexible adhesive tapes used to encircle appendages with pads and bandages.

6. Athletic tape is a strong, sticky tape that provides structural support by wrapping joints and appendages.

Tools and Safety

1. Disposable Gloves - plastic hand covering to protect first aid responders and victims from contaminating or infecting one another
2. Tweezers are tiny, portable instruments that extract fragments, splinters, and other material from wounds.
3. A tourniquet can halt blood flow to extremities in serious injuries so the victim doesn't bleed to death.
4. Injury Shears are strong scissors/shears used to cut fabric, tape, and bandages.
5. Surgery Sponges clean wounds and eliminate fluids such as blood.
6. A pressure cuff is called a blood pressure measuring device.
7. Airways: a plastic holding mechanism for the pharynx's airway used in emergency ventilation
8. Using a CPR mask, a first aid professional can conduct CPR on a victim without contaminating themselves or the responder.
9. A neck brace is a structural tool to stabilize the neck after an injury.
10. Watering Syringe: a syringe used to apply liquids, such as water, to wounds and ailments
11. Security Pins are used to secure cloth to the fabric.

First Aid Material Purchasing

First things first, purchase the necessities and receive training. Continue to learn and gradually improve your resources so that you are prepared. Immediately set aside some money to buy supplies and first aid kits. Once a year, check to see if any have expired. Take them out.

Chapter 2: HOW TO PERFORM A FIRST AID ASSESSMENT

Completing an examination of the situation and the person is crucial if they appear hurt. This enables you to detect potentially fatal illnesses and other health issues promptly so the patient can get treatment as soon as possible.

Here's how to assess a responsive individual for first aid.

Adults' First Aid Assessment

1. Make sure you and the victim are safe in any emergency, and then follow conventional procedures to reduce your risk of infection. Wearing gloves and other personal protection equipment (PPE) is part of this.
2. Send someone to grab the first aid box and an AED, assess the patient's breathing and responsiveness, and activate emergency medical services.
3. Ask for permission before assisting if the person is breathing and responding, then act fast to rule out any potentially fatal conditions.

Assessing First Aid While Awaiting EMS (if available)

1. To obtain further information, consider conducting a secondary assessment while you wait for EMS.
2. Request that the individual explain the issue. To ascertain the possible cause of their symptoms, you might need to inquire about them.
3. Seek jewelry with medical identification. Medical jewelry can send important information if the wearer loses consciousness or becomes unresponsive. Search for a little symbol or tag on a necklace or bracelet containing text about bleeding diseases, food or medication allergies, diabetes, or epilepsy.

4. Examine the person's entire body with your eyes. As a guide, make use of the acronym DOTS. Keep an eye out for open wounds and deformities. Inquire about swelling and tenderness. Assign the proper first aid to any issues that are found.
5. Determine the damage process as best you can. This is how the person's injury was sustained. For instance, they might have been injured by a falling object at work, experienced environmental exposure, or been involved in a bicycle accident. This might assist you in estimating the likelihood and seriousness of injuries.
6. Evaluate the scene's safety, response, breathing, and the efficacy of the first aid administered until EMS or someone with more advanced training steps in to take over.
7. Don't forget to provide any information you've learned from your assessments.

Take a First Aid Course

I will remind you many times in this manual.

Are you familiar with treating severe, potentially fatal bleeding? When someone might have suffered a head, neck, or spinal injury, how should you treat them? How should an impaled object be removed?

Take a First Aid Course

THE RECOVERY POSITION IN FIRST AID

In order to keep a patient still, open their airways, and stop aspiration, first responders adopt the recovery posture. Aspiration happens when a liquid or foreign substance (such as food or vomit) inadvertently gets into the lungs or airways and chokes the victim.

When a person is breathing regularly and has lost consciousness but does not require CPR or chest compressions, they should be placed in the recovery position. In situations like alcohol poisoning, heat stroke, or when a person is unable to remain upright, the position may be used.

In this chapter, we will discuss when it is appropriate to employ the recovery position, how to position the individual correctly, and when it is not.

When to Utilize the Recovery Position

While awaiting additional medical attention, a person with diminished consciousness who is still breathing and does not have any other life-threatening illnesses should be put in the recovery position. Reduced consciousness can take several forms, from somnolence (drowsiness) to coma (unresponsiveness).

If numerous individuals at the scene are seriously injured, first responders will also put someone in the recovery position. The recovery position frees the first responder to tend to other patients who may require more urgent, life-saving care or CPR without having to stay by the side of the person with impaired responsiveness who does not require it.

Conditions in which the recovery position is employed include:

- Heat-related illness
- Toxicology of opioids (overdose)
- Poisoning, particularly poisoning from alcohol

- Respiratory failure
- Following a cardiac arrest, abrupt restoration of circulation

A person shouldn't be put in the recovery position if they are having cardiac arrest, have abnormal breathing, or require chest compressions or CPR. Rather, immediate use of an automated external defibrillator (AED) or chest compressions is recommended.

How to Place Someone in a Recovery Position

Make sure the scene is secure first. If so, determine whether the person is breathing and conscious. You should now search for any further severe injuries, such as neck injuries.

Place the victim in the recovery position while you wait for emergency services if they are breathing but not fully conscious and if there are no additional injuries.

Before placing an unconscious individual in a recovery posture, you must clear their airway if they are not breathing.

To place someone in a position of recovery:

- Next to them, kneel. Check that they are facing upwards and extend their arms and legs straight.
- Fold the arm that is nearest to you across their chest.
- Stretch the arm that is the furthest away from your body in an outward motion.
- At the knee, bend the leg that is nearest to you.
- Using one hand, support the person's neck and head. Roll the person away from you while holding their bent knee.
- To maintain an open and unobstructed airway, tilt the person's head back.

Who Must Not Be Placed in Recovery Position

Although the recovery position is frequently employed in first aid scenarios, there are other circumstances in which it is inappropriate. In certain instances, transferring an individual onto their side or moving them in any way could worsen their injury.

In case the victim has spinal cord, head, or neck injuries, do not place them in the recovery posture. Furthermore, it is not appropriate to employ the recovery position when:

- The individual is going into cardiac arrest
- The patient needs CPR or chest compressions
- The person is exhaling or breathing in agony, which is unnatural

The recovery position might be more detrimental in certain situations. An automated external defibrillator (AED) or cardiopulmonary resuscitation (chest compressions) are instead urgently needed.

For children younger than one, the recovery position is not recommended. Rather, lay the infant across your forearm, face down. Be sure to use your hand to support the baby's head.

The Purpose and Expectations of the Recovery Position

Allowing everything that is regurgitated to drain out of the mouth is the aim of the recovery position. The apex of the trachea (windpipe) and the esophagus (food pipe) are adjacent to each other. Matter that escapes the esophagus has the potential to enter the lungs with ease. This could cause aspiration pneumonia, an infection of the lungs brought on by foreign objects, or it could essentially drown the victim.

The preferred recovery position in the past has been on the left side. However, a recent study indicates that, for the most part, it probably doesn't matter whose side you place the individual on.

Does It Work?

Regretfully, there isn't much data to support the effectiveness or ineffectiveness of the recovery position. This is due to a lack of research to look forward to.

What Science Says

A 2016 research examined the association between the recovery posture and hospital admission in 553 children with loss of consciousness aged 0 to 18. The children who had their caretakers place them in the recovery posture had a lower hospital admission rate, according to the research.

According to different research, if a person going through cardiac arrest is placed in the recovery posture, onlookers might not be aware of when they cease breathing. This can cause the process of performing CPR to take longer.

Additionally, studies have shown that the left-side recovery posture is not well tolerated by patients with congestive heart failure (CHF), a kind of cardiac illness.

The European Resuscitation Council continues to advise placing unconscious people in the recovery position despite the scant evidence, but it also states that vital signs should be regularly observed.

Tips for Assisting Others

The recovery posture can be helpful in some circumstances; however, it might need to be modified depending on the scenario.

Excess dosage

An overdose involves more than just the possibility of aspirating vomit. One may still have undigested capsules in their stomach if they overindulged in tablets. The left-side recovery posture has been shown in studies to potentially reduce the absorption of several medications. Therefore, until assistance arrives, someone who has overdosed can benefit from being placed in the left-side recovery position.

Epilepsy

Prior to putting the patient in the recovery posture, wait until the seizure has ended. If the victim hurt themselves during the seizure or is having difficulty breathing afterward, try to calm him down and keep him from hurting himself.

In addition, in case this is the individual's first seizure or if the episode lasts longer than usual, this can be a critical situation in which to pay more attention. Seeking emergency care is especially necessary in cases of seizures lasting more than five minutes or numerous seizures occurring quickly after one another.

The two most important things to check for after someone receives CPR and starts breathing are if they are continuing breathing and whether any vomit has left anything in their airway. This might entail placing them on their stomach or in the recovery posture.

For many years, the recovery posture has been the accepted position for those who are unconscious. There isn't much proof, though, if it works or doesn't. While some research has shown advantages, others have shown that the recovery posture may hurt patients with congestive heart failure or cause delays in the delivery of CPR.

A person's positioning should be determined by the circumstances. A person who has overdosed on a chemical may be prevented from absorbing it by adopting the recovery posture. Someone who has recently experienced a seizure could additionally find it useful.

RESCUE BREATHING

A person who collapses and loses breathing needs rescue breathing. This chapter is meant to assist those who are not breathing but still have a pulse (their heart is still pumping). In the event that the person is not breathing and is not pulsed, begin cardiopulmonary resuscitation (CPR). If the person's heart is not beating, rescue breathing may be performed in addition to chest compressions during CPR.

This section provides you with an overview of the fundamentals of rescue breathing. It is not meant to serve as a substitute for CPR instruction.

In the following circumstances, rescue breathing could be necessary:

- Severe asthma attack; overdose or poisoning; near drowning; choking; and carbon monoxide poisoning
- You can provide enough oxygen to sustain life by breathing into the lungs of another person, a technique known as rescue breathing. Take immediate action since a lack of oxygen can cause brain damage in as little as three minutes.
- Give one rescue breath every two or three seconds, or around 20 to 30 breaths per minute, if the victim is a baby or kid (age 1 to puberty) and they are not breathing but have a pulse.

If no EMS is available, take the following actions:

- Give one rescue breath every five to six seconds, or around ten to twelve breaths per minute, if the patient is not breathing but is still pulse-free.
- If you feel you are able to perform CPR, start it if the patient has no pulse.
- Protective face mask: A protective face mask is an option. Observe the instructions included with the mask.

Step 1: Let the airway open.

- Place the victim on their back.
- Apply pressure with your hand on the person's forehead. In the same instant, push the chin away from the spine by hooking your fingers beneath it, much like you would when you pull out a drawer. This opens the airway and tilts the head back.
- Lay the person on their back without moving their chin or neck if there is a chance they might have suffered a head, neck, or spine injury.

Step 2: Look for a pulse and breathing

- Observe whether the chest is rising.
- Pay attention to regular breathing—not panting for air.
- Examine for a pulse.

Start mouth-to-mouth breathing using the techniques outlined in Steps 3 through 5 if the patient is not breathing normally but is still breathing.

Step 3: Pinch and seal

Both adults and kids (up to puberty):

- Keep the chin up and the head tilted back.
- With your thumb and first finger, pinch the victim's nostrils together, or adhere to the instructions on your face mask.
- Put your lips over the victim's open mouth if you don't have a barrier to protect them.

Note: You can cover the victim's nose with your lips if they are unable to open their mouth.

Infants (up to age 1):

- Put your mouth or a barrier between the baby's nose and mouth to protect them.

Step 4: Give a life-saving breath

- Both adults and kids (up to puberty):
- Take a single breath into the victim's mouth. When the chest rises, observe it.
- Air enters the person's lungs if their chest elevates.

Infants (up to age 1):

- Instead of taking one big breath, provide two little puffs or breaths of air. Every inhale should take one second.
- If the victim's chest rises, gently puff on them or breathe again into their mouth.
- Tilt the victim's head back and raise their chin if their chest doesn't rise. Next, inhale once again into the victim's mouth.

Chest compressions should be performed; if the chest doesn't rise, look into the mouth for a foreign object. Use your fingers to sweep the lips of anything visible, then take it out. Be cautious not to force the item farther into the throat. Never blindly swipe your finger across someone's mouth.

Step 5. Give more breaths

- Both adults and kids (up to puberty):

Until the victim begins breathing or emergency medical assistance arrives, keep giving one rescue breath every five to six seconds, or around ten to twelve breaths per minute.

Every two minutes, check for a pulse. Start CPR if there is no pulse.

For infants under one-year-old, provide two breaths after thirty chest compressions until the child begins to breathe or until help arrives.

In case of an emergency, it is advisable to be ready. Search online or in your community for lessons provided by the American Red Cross, the American Heart Association, or your neighborhood hospital.

Chapter 3: CPR GUIDE

If someone is not breathing, doing CPR on them can assist in keeping them alive until help arrives. It's critical to understand when and how to do CPR. CPR functions by maintaining a person's blood flow until medical personnel arrive to assist them. The CPR procedures can still save a life, even for those without first aid expertise.

CPR can increase or even triple a person's chances of survival if it is performed as soon as their heart stops beating.

CPR Procedures: Fast Reference

When an adult is not breathing or is only intermittently gasping, as well as when they are not reacting to questions or shoulder taps, perform CPR.

When a child or newborn is not breathing regularly and not reacting, do CPR on them.

After ensuring that everyone is secure, carry out the following fundamental CPR procedures:

Once the patient is on their back, clear their airway.

Check for breathing. Start CPR if they are not breathing.

Do thirty compressions on the chest.

Take two rescue breaths.

Continue doing this until an automated external defibrillator (AED) or ambulance comes.

Continue reading for more thorough instructions on how to administer CPR to adults, kids, and newborns.

Step-by-step CPR

The preparation stage and the CPR stage are the two primary phases of CPR.

Use the following preparatory measures before administering CPR to an adult:

Step 1: Look for someone who can help you or keep the situation under control.

First, look around the area for anything that can endanger you, such as falling masonry, traffic, or fire. Check the person after that. Do they require aid? Shake hands with them and ask, "Are you okay?"

Before doing CPR, if they are not responding, look for someone who can help you. Ask a passerby to look for an AED machine if at all feasible. These are available for use in workplaces and several other public facilities.

Step 2: Turn the patient over onto their back and clear their airway.

Gently lay the individual on their back, then bend down to squat next to their chest. Raise their chin to gently slant their head back.

Examine their mouth for any blockages, such as food particles or vomit. If there is a loose blockage, remove it. If it is not loose, trying to grasp it may push it farther into the airway.

Step 3: Check for breathing

Place your ear next to the person's mouth and listen for no more than 10 seconds. If you do not hear breathing or you only hear occasional gasps, begin CPR.

Don't attempt CPR on someone unconscious but still breathing. Instead, put them in the recovery posture if they don't appear to have a spinal injury. Continue to keep an eye on their breathing, and if they stop, do CPR.

Step 4: Do thirty compressions on the chest

Clasp your hands together by putting one on top of the other. Firmly press in the middle of the chest, just below the nipples, using the heel of your palms and straight elbows.

Press down at least two inches. Compress their chest at a rate of at least 100 times per minute. In between compressions, allow the chest to expand entirely.

Step 5: Perform two rescue breaths

Tilt their head back slightly and elevate their chin, making sure their mouth is clean. To make their chest rise, pinch their nose shut, cover their entire lips with yours, and blow.

Retilt their head if, upon taking a first breath, their chest does not lift. The person could be choking if their chest does not rise with a second breath.

Step 6: Carry On

Continue doing two rescue breaths and 30 chest compressions until the individual begins to breathe on their own or aid comes. Continue administering CPR until the AED is ready for use in the event that one comes.

CPR for Young People and Babies

The procedures for doing CPR on toddlers and newborns differ slightly from those for adults, as shown below.

Take the following preparatory actions before administering CPR to a baby or child:

Step 1: Look for someone who can help you or keep the situation under control.

Start by looking around for anything that could endanger you. Check the youngster or newborn again to determine whether they require assistance. Give a youngster a shoulder tap and shout, "Are you okay?" To find out if a baby responds, flick the bottom of their foot.

Give the youngster two minutes of attention if you are the only one with them and they are not reacting. If someone is observing, ask them to support you.

Ask a passerby to look for an AED machine if at all feasible. Typically, these are located in offices and other public buildings.

Step 2. Lay them flat on their back with their airways open.

Gently lay the baby or toddler on their back, then bend down to squat next to their chest. Raise their chin to gently cock their head back.

Let their mouth open. Look for any blockages, such as food or vomit. Remove it if it's loose. Avoid touching it if it is not loose, as this might cause it to become lodged further in their airways.

Step 3: Make sure they're breathing

Listen to them for around ten seconds by putting your ear near their mouth. Start doing CPR if they are not breathing or are just occasionally gasping.

Since infants typically breathe on a periodic basis, changes in their breathing patterns are natural.

Continue to keep an eye on their respiration, and if they stop, do CPR.

CPR Procedures

To do CPR on a kid or newborn, use these steps:

Step 1: Inhale twice to save yourself.

Give the kid or newborn two rescue breaths while tilting their head back and lifting their chin if they are not breathing.

Pinch a child's nose shut and cover it with your mouth. Twice inhale into their mouth.

To make a baby's chest rise, cover their mouth and nose with yours and blow for one second. Next, give two rescue breaths.

Start chest compressions if they are still not responding.

Step 2: Do thirty compressions on the chest.

Be on your knees by the baby or youngster.

Use one of your hands to a youngster. Lay the heel of your hand between and just below their nipples at their sternum, which is located in the middle of their chest. At least 100 times per minute, apply forceful, rapid pressure to a depth of about 2 inches, or one-third the depth of the chest.

If the baby is little, use two fingers. Put your fingers between and just below their nipples in the middle of their chest. Execute thirty rapid compressions that are about 1.5 inches deep.

Step 3: Repeat.

Rescue breathing and chest compressions should be repeated until the youngster begins to breathe on their own or assistance comes.

When Not To Do CPR and When To

When a person is not breathing, CPR can help save their brain.

When an adult is not breathing at all, perform CPR. If a kid or newborn is not breathing regularly, do CPR on them. If you speak to or tap an adult or kid who is not reacting, you should always do CPR.

Giving CPR can guarantee that blood rich in oxygen reaches the brain in cases where the person is not breathing. This is crucial because, without oxygen, a person might pass away in less than eight minutes or suffer irreversible brain damage.

If someone stops breathing in any of the following situations, they might need CPR:

- a heart attack or cardiac arrest
- choking
- traffic accident
- drowning
- asphyxiation
- overdosing on drugs
- poisoning
- cigarette ingestion
- electrical shock
- sudden infant death syndrome suspicions

Perform CPR only if the adult is not breathing or, in the case of children and babies, if their respiration is irregular and their blood is not flowing. For this reason, before beginning CPR, be sure the patient is not responding to any physical or verbal cues to stop.

CPR is a first aid technique that can save lives. It can greatly increase someone's chances of survival if they have a heart attack or become unconscious after an injury or accident.

Depending on the person's age—infant, child, or adult—different stages apply. The fundamental sequence of rescue breaths and chest compressions won't change, though.

Apply CPR only after an adult has lost consciousness. Prior to beginning CPR, ascertain whether the patient reacts to spoken or tactile cues.

Chapter 4: BITES AND STINGS

Not every sting or bite is the same. The sort of species that bit or stung you will determine what kind of medical attention and first aid you require. Certain animals can do more harm than others. Additionally, some people are more susceptible to extreme reactions due to allergies.

Here's how to identify and handle symptoms of bug, spider, and snake bites and stings.

Insects

Almost everyone has experienced an insect bite or sting at some point in their lives. Insect stings and bites typically result in a little reaction, regardless of the bug that bit you—a wasp, fly, bee, mosquito, or another kind of insect. When an insect injects venom or other proteins into you or ingests them through their saliva, your body responds. This can lead to the following symptoms to appear where the bite or sting occurred:

- Redness
- Pain
- Swelling
- Itching

The kind of bug that bites or stings you will determine how severe your symptoms are. Insect bites or stings can also cause severe allergic reactions in certain people. Allergies in bees and wasps are very prevalent. One sign of a severe allergic response is:

- Hives
- Nausea and vomiting
- Stomach cramps
- Shock
- Swelling of the face, lip, or throat

Search for a local emergency services if you or someone you know starts to exhibit these symptoms soon after being bitten or stung by an insect. Anaphylaxis is the term for a severe allergic response that affects many different regions of the body. If not treated right away, it can turn fatal.

See your doctor about allergy testing if you've ever experienced a severe response to a bite or sting from an insect. If your doctor has determined that you have a severe allergy, they should give you epinephrine. You can inject the drug into the muscle of your outer thigh using an EpiPen® or other preloaded epinephrine auto-injector. It works fast to increase heart rate, elevate blood pressure, and lessen airway edema. It is important that you always have it on you, particularly while you are outside in places where insects can be present.

First Aid Procedures

Help someone seek emergency medical assistance and proceed as outlined in the next section if they exhibit symptoms of a severe allergic reaction. Treat any mild symptoms at the bite or sting site if they don't exhibit any indicators of a serious response.

If the stinger of the bug is still stuck in their flesh, remove it with a gentle scrape of a flat-edged instrument over their skin, like a credit card. Squeezing the stinger with tweezers might cause it to emit more venom, so avoid doing so.

Use soap and water to clean the bite area.

For around ten minutes at a time, apply an ice pack or cold compress to the affected region to aid with discomfort and swelling. To protect their skin, wrap any ice or ice packs in a fresh towel.

To aid with itching and discomfort relief, use calamine lotion or a paste made of baking soda and water to the region several times a day. One kind of antihistamine cream is calamine lotion.

Treatment for a Severe Allergic Response in an Emergency

If you think someone could be experiencing a serious allergic reaction:

- Ask someone to look for a treatment kit for allergic reactions in a health care facility where there may still be staff or materials stored.
- Find out whether the person has an auto-injector for epinephrine with them. If so, get it for them and assist them in using it in accordance with the instructions on the label.
- Urge them to remain motionless, lie down quietly with their legs propped up, and maintain their composure. In order to prevent choking and to let the vomit drain, flip them onto their side if they begin to vomit.
- Start CPR if they lose consciousness and cease breathing. Keep doing so until medical assistance comes.
- If possible, avoid applying a tourniquet to aggravate the situation. Moreover, you ought to refrain from offering them any food or beverages.

Spiders

The majority of spider bites are not too harmful. You can have symptoms similar to an insect bite or sting anywhere from a few hours to a day following your bite. At the biting site, you could feel:

- redness
- swelling
- discomfort
- itching

Certain spider species, such as brown recluse and black widow spiders, might have greater detrimental effects. Knowing what to look for makes it simple to distinguish between the two species.

Black widow spiders usually measure around 1/2 inch when fully developed. They have a red hourglass marking on the bottom of their belly, and their body is black. Additionally, some black widow spiders have red patches on the top abdomen surface and red bars running across the underside.

The poison of black widow spiders disrupts your neurological system. You could experience excruciating agony at the bite location for a few hours after being bitten. Other symptoms, including chills, fever, stomach discomfort, nausea, and vomiting, are also possible.

Compared to black widow spiders, brown recluse spiders are bigger when fully matured. They are around one inch long. Their hues range from dark brown to a yellowish tan. On their upper torso, they have a marking like a violin, with the neck of the instrument pointing in the direction of their back and the base of the instrument looking toward their head.

Skin injury results from bites by brown recluse spiders. After being bitten, you will notice severe pain and redness at the bite site within eight hours. A blister will eventually form. Your skin will develop a deep ulcer that can get infected when the blister bursts. Additionally, you can have symptoms including nausea, rash, and fever.

First Aid Procedures

If you believe someone has been bitten by a black widow or brown recluse spider, assist them in getting medical attention right away and take the actions outlined in this section. If not, handle their spider bite the same way you would other bug stings and bites:

Use soap and water to clean the bite area.

For approximately ten minutes, apply an ice pack or cold compress to the affected region to aid with pain and swelling. To protect their skin, wrap any ice or ice packs in a fresh towel.

To aid with itching and pain relief, use calamine lotion or a paste made of baking soda and water on the damaged area. One popular antihistamine cream is calamine lotion.

Emergency Treatment For a Brown Recluse or Black Widow Spider Bite

In the event that you believe a black widow or brown recluse spider has bitten someone:

Use soap and water to clean the bite area.

In order to stop the poison from spreading, urge them to stay still and composed.

On the bite site, use an ice pack or cold compress. To protect their skin, wrap ice or ice packs in a clean towel.

Take a photo or description of the spider that bit them if it is safe to do so. This can assist healthcare providers in diagnosing it and selecting the best course of action.

Never use a tourniquet.

Don't provide them with any food or liquids.

Snakes

Although most snake species are benign, some can bite humans and cause severe injury. In the United States, common poisonous snake species include:

- cotton head
- cottonmouth
- coral rattlesnakes

Depending on the kind of snake, there might be a wide range of symptoms from a bite. They may consist of:

- fragility
- fainting
- dizziness
- convulsions
- sick stomach
- vomiting, diarrhea, and fast heartbeat
- decrease in muscular coordination
- edema around the biting site

A poisonous snake bite is an emergency. Early intervention can reduce symptoms and accelerate healing.

Treatment With First Aid for Minor Bites

Assist the victim of a snake bite in receiving immediate medical attention and proceed with the following session's instructions if you believe the snake may have been poisonous. In the event that you are certain the snake was not poisonous, attend to any bleeding and other symptoms in the bite area:

Apply pressure to the area with a clean towel or gauze until the bleeding stops.

Use soap and water to clean the area.

Use a cream containing antibiotics to help prevent infection.

To protect the wound as it heals, cover it with gauze or a sterile bandage.

Assist the victim in receiving immediate medical attention if they are bleeding heavily. Keep adding fresh layers of cloth or gauze to the bleeding region over previously applied layers that are completely saturated with blood. Eliminating older layers can worsen the bleeding.

Treatment for Poisonous Snake Bites in an Emergency

Should you believe that a poisonous snake has bitten an individual:

Urge them to settle down, be motionless, and keep their composure. The poison can get into their body more quickly if they move.

Tight clothes or jewelry should be taken from the area around the bite since edema might develop there.

Treat them for shock if they have pale, clammy skin, weakness, disorientation, shortness of breath, or elevated heart rate. To keep them warm, give them a blanket or an additional layer of clothes.

Take a picture or a description of the snake that bit them if it is safe to do so. This can assist medical personnel in identifying the snake and choosing the best course of action.

To stop things from becoming worse, don't:

Put yourself in danger by attempting to catch the snake, then clean the bite site since the snake's remaining venom can assist medical personnel in determining the kind of snake and the best course of action.

Apply a cold compress to the bite site; elevate the portion that was bitten above the level of the heart; cut or suction the bite site; and provide the victim with food or liquids.

Provide any painkillers to the patient.

Most individuals have, at some point in their life, been bitten or stung by insects, spiders, or snakes. Simple first aid care is typically sufficient for minor bites and stings. Address any little bleeding, swelling, soreness, or itching in the affected region.

As soon as you believe someone is experiencing a serious response from a bite or sting, assist them in getting medical treatment. A bite or sting may cause a severe allergic reaction in people with specific sensitivities. Certain animals, such as poisonous snakes, brown recluse spiders, and black widow spiders, can cause a great deal of harm. You can protect others and yourself by being ready for any emergency.

Chapter 5: CHOKING

Choking can occur when food particles or other foreign objects become stuck in the airway. When someone chokes, oxygen cannot reach the brain and lungs. If oxygen is not given to the brain for more than four minutes, brain damage or even death may result. Everyone should be aware of the signs of choking and know how to respond to it in both private and public settings. Experts recommend treating a choking adult or kid older than one year old using back strikes and abdominal thrusts.

How Can I Avoid Becoming Choked?

Adult choking can be avoided by using the following safety precautions:

Cut food into little bits.

Chew meals properly and slowly, particularly if you're wearing dentures.

While chewing and swallowing, avoid laughing and talking.

Limit your alcohol intake both before and during meals.

Children shouldn't choke on objects if you take these precautions:

Especially with smaller children, keep little toys and things like marbles, beads, thumbtacks, latex balloons, money, and other items out of reach.

When children have food or toys in their mouths, stop them from playing, walking, or running.

Foods that are prone to being stuck in the throat shouldn't be given to kids under the age of four. For example, hot dogs, almonds, cheese or meat pieces, grapes, hard candies, popcorn, raw carrots, and peanut butter chunks.

Watch over little children at mealtimes.

Stop older siblings from giving a small kid a toy or food that might be harmful.

What Is the Recommended Choking First Aid Technique?

If a person or kid over one-year-old is cognizant and choking on food or a foreign item, a series of back blows and abdominal thrusts beneath the diaphragm are recommended. A person who is choking is unable to breathe, speak, or cough due to an obstruction in their airway. Air cannot pass through. The obstruction of the airway can result in death or a loss of consciousness. Be careful not to force yourself when performing the abdominal thrusts to avoid hurting your internal organs or ribs. Use chest compressions if the victim is unconscious.

First, deliver five back strikes in succession.

Lean the individual forward gently, if you can, until their upper body is parallel to the ground. To provide support, place one arm over the person's chest. Bend over the individual if they are a child.

Five fast thumps (back strikes) between the person's shoulder blades should be delivered with the heel of your free hand.

After that, give five abdominal thrusts. Pushes from the abdomen raise the diaphragm. They expel sufficient air from the lungs to produce a fake cough. This cough facilitates air passage via the windpipe, forcing the blockage out of the mouth and airway:

Grab the person's waist with your arm.

Put one closed hand below the rib cage and above the navel or belly button.

With your other hand, make a fist. Five fast times, pull the clinched hand straight, forcefully, backward, and upward under the rib cage.

Give chest thrusts if the person is obese or in the latter stages of pregnancy.

Continue abdominal thrusts and back blows until the blockage is removed, the patient loses consciousness, or advanced life support is made available. In either scenario, the patient has to be seen as quickly as possible by a medical professional.

Thrusts on oneself are an option if you find yourself suffocating and alone. Alternatively, you can press your upper abdomen up against a chair's back or a counter's edge.

Back strikes and abdominal thrusts should only be performed in true emergencies, when it is certain that the individual is choking, in order to limit potential injury. Only use this technique on adults and kids older than one-year-old.

For newborns under one-year-old, a different technique is employed. Have a conversation with your child's healthcare practitioner about the proper first aid procedure for choking.

How Can I Get Properly Trained To Assist Someone Who Is Choking?

It's easy to learn how to use abdominal thrusts and back strikes. Classes on first aid and cardiopulmonary resuscitation (CPR) frequently cover it. Get in touch with the American Heart Association or American Red Cross branch in your area. Please get in touch with your nearby hospital or healthcare center for further information and a class schedule.

Chapter 6: BURNS

A burn injury is a tissue damage caused by fires or prolonged exposure to sunlight or any other kind of radiation, as well as contact with hot surfaces or chemicals. Burns can be first, second, or third degree.

First Aid Measures for First-Degree Burns or Small Burns

Dos (√):

To reduce discomfort, apply cold running water to the burnt area for ten to fifteen minutes, making sure it's not freezing.

Take off any jewelry, watches, belts, or other accessories, and swiftly and carefully take off any shoes or clothing before the region expands.

To lessen the chance of infection, cover the burn with a cold, clean cloth or a moist, sterile bandage.

If you need to, use medicines to ease your discomfort.

If the burns are serious and cover a significant portion of the body, or if you have increasing pain, redness, or swelling, or if you suspect an infection, get medical attention.

Don'ts (X):

Don't try touching the blister bubbles resulting from the burn.

Use of butter, toothpaste, ointments, or other burn cures is not advised.

Ice shouldn't be applied immediately to the burnt area.

First Aid Procedures for Burns of the Second Degree

Dos (√):

Protect the burnt individual against more injury.

Take off belts, rings, and other constricting objects, especially from the vicinity of burnt regions like the neck.

If you need to, use medicines to ease your discomfort.

Use a cold, clean towel or a moist, sterile bandage to cover the burn.

Seal blisters that have erupted using a clean, dry bandage.

Don'ts (X):

Don't remove burned clothing stuck to the skin.

Never use an adhesive bandage to hide a burn.

Larger burnt body parts should not be submerged in cold water as this might result in shock.

Ice shouldn't be applied immediately to the burnt area.

Use of butter, toothpaste, ointments, or other burn cures is not advised.

Refrain from touching the burn-related blister bubbles.

Do not apply thin cotton to the burnt area, as it can lead to skin irritation.

Third-Degree Burns

These burns damage all layers of skin, penetrate the fat layer, and occasionally even reach the underlying muscle tissue. They are regarded as the most severe type of burns.

Dos (√):

Perform the following actions until medical aid is available:

Assess the patient's respiration and other vital indicators.

Keep the burn victim away from heat sources, smoke, and combustible materials to prevent more injury.

If at all feasible, raise the burnt region above the patient's heart level.

Use a cold, clean towel or a moist, sterile bandage to cover the burn.

Don'ts (X):

Don't remove burned clothing stuck to the skin.

Larger burnt body parts shouldn't be submerged in cold water since this might result in shock or an abrupt drop in body temperature.

Never use an adhesive bandage to hide a burn.

Use of butter, toothpaste, ointments, or other burn cures is not advised.

Avoid using thin cotton on the burnt area as it may cause skin irritation.

Following hospital burn treatment, the skin needs extra attention at home, which includes:

Bathing: you can still take your regular shower and wash your hair; however, soaking in a bathtub is not recommended. It's also crucial to check the water's temperature before stepping into the shower since freshly healed skin is susceptible to injury from extremely hot or cold water. Don't massage the skin too hard, either. It's important that you follow any directions your healthcare professional gives you regarding taking medicine and dressing the wound before taking a bath.

Dry Skin: skin dryness is caused by damage to the skin's fat layer. Until this layer starts to function normally, you'll need to use moisturizers and lotions. Try to avoid skin moisturizers that contain lanolin and alcohol, as they tend to create blisters in the healed skin.

Itchiness: this feeling is typically present in conjunction with dry, scaly, and healed skin. Scratching the afflicted region should be avoided as this might destroy the freshly developed fragile skin layers. Applying moisturizers or lotions as required is advised instead. Your doctor could suggest a prescription to assist in reducing acute itching if you are experiencing this issue.

Bruises: after the burns have healed, each person will experience a new layer of skin that is thinner, more sensitive, and fragile than the rest of their body for a variable amount of time. It could take a few months for some people and a year or longer for others. These regions are prone to bruising; thus, it's important to protect them from burns and sharp objects to prevent bruises. Additionally, as your body needs time to heal and develop pressure-resistant skin fully, you should refrain from wearing tight clothing or shoes that might create blisters.

Blisters: blisters are not to be concerned about; they are a frequent side effect of friction, rubbing, or brushing against things throughout the healing process. Blisters seem to occur on certain persons more easily than on others. As the new skin thickens, this propensity lessens. It is best to see your healthcare practitioner about how to treat blisters if they develop.

Feeling Cold: your newly thinned skin will be more susceptible to freezing conditions. You can feel a little tingling and numbness in the cold, especially in your hands and feet. The better your skin gets, the less noticeable this sensation will become. By dressing warmly and limiting your time outside in the cold, you can lessen your suffering. It is advisable to shield your skin for a minimum of a year.

Sunshine Sensitivity: your recently healed skin is more susceptible to the sun's rays and might burn more intensely in short amounts of time. It is thus advised to cover the impacted region with lightweight clothing in order to protect it. If you have burns on your face or neck, you can also wear a large cap. It is crucial to consistently apply sunscreen to the impacted region, particularly in the summer. After at least a year of constant use, you can start to assess the sensitivity of your skin to sunlight.

Skin Appearance: during the healing phase, some scarring and alterations in the skin's appearance are normal.

Skin Discoloration: the typical healing process is what causes the skin discoloration you notice in your healed skin. It doesn't matter if it looks pink, brown, or grayish—this is normal. Each person experiences discoloration differently based on the inherent hue of their skin. In a few months, second-degree burns may regain their natural color. Conversely, third-degree burns could take a lot longer, and burns that are deeper might even result in some permanent discoloration.

Discoloration of extremities: walking or moving your arms may cause some discoloration if the burn is close to your arms or legs. It could be beneficial to sit with your feet elevated on a chair to assist in easing this leg pain. If you walk instead of standing still, you might find that you are more comfortable. Long periods of inactivity cause the blood in your legs and feet to pool, which can result in edema and discoloration. Moderate exercise will also help your circulation. On your subsequent appointment, you should let your healthcare practitioner know if this issue persists.

Scarring: discoloration is generally associated with scarring. At first, it's quite impossible to predict how much of the scarring will last. There are certain persons who are more likely to scar. Each person experiences scarring differently and at varying degrees of damage. First-degree burn scars and mild second-degree burns may go away in a few months. Deep second and third-degree burns, however, might require at least two years to heal. In most cases, scars deepen over time. They will appear at their worst four to eight months after the burn, and then they will progressively get better over time.

Chapter 7: SPRAINS AND STRAINS

An injury to the capsule and ligaments at a joint in the body is called a sprain. Damage to tendons or muscles is called a strain. Immediate treatment of sprains or strains includes protection, optimal loading, ice, compression and elevation. It is recommended that you have ongoing therapy and monitoring before returning to normal activities.

There are two types of soft tissue injuries: acute and chronic. The kind of tissue and extent of the injury, the type of therapy received, prior injuries, the patient's age and general health, and other variables all affect how quickly an injury heals.

Why Do People Get Sprains and Strains?

Fiber bundles make up soft tissue structures. Specialized cells found in muscles and tendons track the amount of contraction and stretch. Soft contractions are the general mechanism used by muscles and tendons to prevent overstretching. Nevertheless, abrupt twists or jolts can apply more force than the tissue can withstand, causing the fibers to rip or burst. The swelling is brought on by bleeding from ruptured blood vessels.

Soft tissue injuries, such as those to tendons and ligaments, can develop gradually or suddenly. An acute soft tissue injury is a sudden injury that is typically associated with a particular occurrence. This indicates that it happened during the last 72 hours. An injury commonly known as a chronic soft tissue injury has persisted for three months or more. These are frequently brought on by improper loading, also known as "overuse," in which the tissue's capability is overwhelmed by the physical demands made on it.

A Sprain

Ligaments are strong bands of connective tissue that support and stabilize joints. Joint capsules do this job. A membrane containing lubricating synovial fluid surrounds the whole joint, providing additional impact protection and joint nourishment. An injury known as a sprain is one in which there is ripping of the ligaments, the joint capsule, or both. Sprains frequently occur in the thumb, ankle, and knee.

Stresses

Tendons are the connective tissue that anchors muscles to joints. A strain is an injury to these tendons or the muscles themselves. The groin, hamstring, and calf are common locations for strains.

Signs of Strained and Sprained Muscles

The following are possible signs of a sprain or strain:

- swelling
- pain
- stiffness
- decreased functional efficiency

Sprain and strain severity levels: acute soft tissue injuries can be categorized based on their level of severity.

Grade I: function and strength are mostly unaltered, mild discomfort and swelling are present, and a small number of fibers are torn.

Grade II: there is some loss of function and strength, a painful, swollen location, and a moderate percentage of ripped fibers.

Grade III: There may be a total rupture of the soft tissue, resulting in a significant loss of strength and function. Getting a medical opinion for these injuries is advised.

Emergency Care for Sprains and Strains

Acute sprains or strains should be treated right away using the following advice:

- Quit what you're doing.
- Let the wounded area rest.
- Put icepacks on the area for 20 minutes every 2 hours, separated from the skin by wet toweling.
- Firmly compress or bandage the damaged area, encircling it from below to above.
- Whenever possible, elevate the wounded region above the level of the heart.
- Within the first 72 hours following the injury, stay away from heat, alcohol, jogging, and massage of the injured region since these activities might exacerbate swelling.
- In the event that symptoms worsen during the first twenty-four hours, consult a medic (if available in your scenario) for further testing.

Overuse Accidents

Anyone who spends hours each day at a computer keyboard or who is an athlete or participant in regular sports might get an overuse injury.

If an overuse injury is not appropriately treated, it frequently gets worse over time. Several injuries can cause discomfort during action and potentially discomfort at rest. Poor technique, structural abnormalities, and too frequent exercise without adequate recuperation time are all contributing reasons for overuse injuries. Every treatment strategy must take into account the injury's natural course and make adjustments for any contributory circumstances.

It is crucial to implement a rehabilitation program that gradually "reloads" the wounded region. In order to observe progress from overuse injuries, patients and clinicians must be patient and committed to the rehabilitation process, which might take some time.

Taking Care of Sprains and Strains

Depending on the degree of the sprain or strain, any further injuries or problems, including weakness, stiffness, impaired balance or function, and the person's overall health, the majority of soft tissue injuries require a few weeks to recover. To aid in a quicker recovery, it's critical to receive the appropriate care as soon as possible following the accident. If the pain and swelling don't go down after a few days, or if you don't have complete function in the affected region, consult a medic (if available in your scenario).

Treatment options might be:

Exercises to support healing, strength, and flexibility; manual methods, including massage and mobilization; electrotherapy; painkillers (consult your doctor or pharmacist before taking any medications, as they can occasionally interfere with the healing process for soft tissue injuries); gradually restoring activities to normal levels.

Surgery may be necessary to repair severely damaged tissue when it has totally burst. Significant therapy is necessary to restore strength and function in grade III injuries that were surgically corrected. The medium-to-long-term functional results for treatment of a grade III injury are comparable whether you have surgery or a period of immobilization and physical therapy.

Chapter 8: DISLOCATIONS

When the bones of a person's joint are forced or knocked out of their normal position, it results in a dislocation. The top of an individual's arm bone, for example, fits into a joint at the shoulder. A dislocated shoulder occurs if it snaps or falls out of that exact joint.

In a similar vein, dislocations can occur in the ankle, knee, shoulder, or hip. A human's skeleton includes joints, which are places where two bones converge.

The bodily tissues around a joint can get torn and strained by dislocation. They are difficult to utilize in the afflicted joint in addition to being painful. It is also able to result in a bone moving to an unnatural location, creating a critical medical hazard.

If a dislocation is not correctly or quickly treated, it might harm a person's ligaments, blood vessels, or nerves.

Dislocation Types

Generally, a person's dislocation is categorized based on how much their joint bones can move. They come in two varieties:

A partial or total dislocation: When the bones of a joint are fully forced out of or separated from their original position, it is known as a total dislocation.

Subluxation: Partial dislocation is another term for subluxation. It describes a situation in which something pulls on a joint while the bones are still partially in contact.

What Are The Signs And Symptoms of a Dislocation?

The history will also point to a dislocation in addition to the physical signs and symptoms, such as the patient's recent fall and decreased range of motion in a specific joint. Most of the time, there will be noticeable swelling and discomfort in the afflicted joint, especially when pressure is applied.

Because of the laxity of the muscles and supporting tissues, certain dislocations, particularly those in individuals who have had several recurrent dislocations at the same joint, may manifest with minor discomfort.

Age is the main factor that determines a patient's risk of dislocating their joint again; young individuals (younger than 20) have a 90 percent or greater risk of dislocating their shoulder again. There is a decreased possibility of re-dislocation as the patient ages.

Dislocations and subluxations can cause the following symptoms:

Injuries may include discomfort, swelling, deformity of the dislocated region, trouble moving or utilizing the damaged part normally, warmth, bruising, or redness in the affected area.

Since the blood supply to joints is fairly restricted, swelling related to dislocations is usually not particularly severe. The patella, or kneecap, is an exception to this rule because of the popliteal artery's proximity and the blood vessel's robust attachments to the femur and tibia.

Dislocation Risk Factors

Anyone who falls or experiences any other type of trauma might have a dislocation. However, elderly individuals are more vulnerable to dislocations if they have an involuntary tendency to fall more frequently. Unsupervised play by children can also cause disruptions, particularly if the place isn't childproofed. Participating in strenuous activities like contact sports also increases the chance of dislocations.

How Long Does It Take to Recuperate From a Dislocation?

Every dislocation has a different healing time depending on the joint that was dislocated and whether the person has any other injuries. The majority of people recover after a few weeks.

However, other joints, like the hips, might take years to fully heal and require surgery. A dislocated finger, on the other hand, can heal in around three weeks. Always get medical advice on how long it will take for a dislocation to recover.

Suppose a person returns to playing sports or doing heavy workouts while the joint hasn't healed. Find out how long they have to wait following the event before they can get back to physical activities like sports or exercise.

How Can a Dislocation Be Prevented?

Dislocations typically result from unforeseeable incidents. Nonetheless, there are a few things to keep in mind to keep yourself as safe as possible when participating in strenuous activities like sports:

- Put on the appropriate safety equipment.
- In the event that you get joint discomfort during or after physical activity, stop playing or exercising.
- Stretch thoroughly before engaging in any exercise or sports.
- After the workout, let your body calm down before performing your post-workout stretches.
- Make sure your body has adequate time to relax and recuperate following an exercise.
- Generally speaking, the following advice can aid in avoiding dislocations:
- Every time you go up and down stairs, utilize the handrails.
- Always keep a first aid kit within reach whenever possible.
- Avoid using throw rugs.
- Keep an eye out for electrical wires covering your floor.

- Avoid using furniture like chairs or tables as a means of access or to remove items from shelves.

The following are some child prevention strategies:

- Make your house secure and childproof.
- Ensure that gates are on your staircases.
- Monitor your children, especially when they're playing.

What Typical Issues Can Result From a Dislocation?

Frequently, a dislocation might result in further difficulties. Some occur in the initial hours or days following the dislocation, while others take longer to manifest. The following are the problems linked to dislocations.

Fractures

Fractures may also result from an injury that produces a dislocation. Rarely, fractures cause the surrounding muscles to enlarge to the point where the blood supply to the injured limb is restricted or obstructed.

If the blood supply isn't replenished promptly, the limb can turn blue, and the tissues within could suffer injury.

Nerve Injury

A person's nerves can frequently get strained or damaged after a dislocation. In these kinds of circumstances, crushed nerves might be far more harmful than damaged ones. Rarely, a patient can additionally have nerve tears, which do not mend on their own.

Tears in the nerve are repaired by surgery; not all nerve injuries recover fully.

Bleeding

The dislocation can cause internal bleeding if it is extremely painful or severe. If the displaced bone impacts the patient's skin, they might experience external bleeding after the procedure.

Contractions

Wounds can occur from a displaced joint that causes the skin to rip. Osteomyelitis, or infection-related bone inflammation, might result from the wounds becoming infected and spreading to the patient's bone.

How are Dislocations Diagnosed?

Someone has to be transported to the hospital right away if they believe they have experienced a dislocation. When patients go to the hospital, they have to go through a physical examination where their joints and the surrounding tissues are checked.

The medic will examine them to see if there is any damage to their skin or circulation in that location. The victim might be put through the following tests:

- CT scan
- MRI
- X-ray
- Ultrasound

Ways to Handle Dislocations

Depending on the joint that has been dislocated and the severity of the patient's condition, several treatments are given for dislocations. The initial course of therapy for dislocation is called the RICE approach, and it involves rest, ice, compression, and elevation.

The following are some possible therapy options if the joint fails to return to its native position:

Using the manipulation technique, medical professionals can realign a patient's joint. To facilitate the surgery and relax the muscles around the joint, the patient is given an anesthetic or sedative.

Medication: After the joint is moved, most patients have no discomfort. If they're still in agony, though, he can take a muscle relaxant or painkiller.

Immobilization: Before a patient's joint heals to its natural position, a cast or sling might be required to be worn for a few weeks. It stops the joint from moving and permits full healing of the affected region.

Surgery: Only when an expert cannot realign a patient's bones or when the patient has suffered damage to their blood vessels or nerves due to a dislocation surgery is necessary. Treating a dislocated shoulder also frequently involves surgery.

Rehabilitation: After the patient's joint has been realigned and they are instructed to take off the sling, the rehabilitation phase begins. After a dislocation, rehabilitation aids in the joint's progressive strengthening.

While each dislocation heals differently, most recover fully. The likelihood that the patient might get more injuries is decreased when care is provided appropriately and promptly.

However, victims must keep in mind that dislocating a joint increases the likelihood that they'll dislocate it again. Thus, to protect oneself against more dislocations, safety measures should be taken, and protective gear should be used.

Chapter 9: HEAD INJURY

Many times, when we consider head injuries, we consider stressful experiences such as auto accidents or sports-related injuries. However, what about routine tasks that put us at risk for a head injury?

A brain injury, regrettably, is not something that should be treated lightly. Understanding the warning signs and symptoms of a brain injury, as well as what to do if you sustain one, is crucial.

A Head Injury: What Is It?

Any damage that causes trauma to the brain is considered a head injury. This can involve harm to the brain, skull, scalp, or other head components. Mild, moderate, and severe head injuries are all possible. They might happen gradually, such as a fall, or easily, like in an automobile accident.

Another name for some brain traumas is concussions. A hit to the head or a sudden shock to the body that causes the brain to move about inside the skull is the typical cause of concussions. This could result in brain damage, and symptoms include headache, nausea, dizziness, and disorientation. The majority of concussion victims recover in a few days with rest and no more medical care.

Serious consequences might come from moderate to severe brain traumas, necessitating hospitalization. These wounds can result in oedema (swelling of the brain) or hemorrhage (bleeding of the brain). They can also end up in brain injury such as fractures to the skull. The quality of life and cognitive function could be negatively impacted for a long time by moderate to severe head injuries.

Signs of Brain Damage

Look for indications of a concussion or a more serious head injury if you believe someone has had a head injury.

The following are indicators that someone might have had a brain injury:

- Have they gone unconscious?
- Did they throw up?
- If so, how many times did they throw up?
- Did they feel sleepy?
- Do they not hear you when you speak to them?
- Does anybody have memory loss? Loss of location, time, and orientation? A very small youngster obviously might not be able to respond to those queries.
- Any disruption to vision? Double or blurry vision?
- Are the sizes of the pupils the same?
- Do the arms and legs feel weak?
- Were they bleeding because of anything trapped in their skull or something else?
- Is there a bruise or a big lump?
- Have they had a seizure fit or convulsion?
- Any discharge or bleeding from the nose or ears.
- A lack of coordination and awkwardness.
- A chronic headache that is unresponsive to paracetamol.
- Coughing or difficulty swallowing.
- Anxiety due to noise.
- Slurred words.

Make immediate contact with emergency services if the person exhibits any of these signs or symptoms following a fall or other head injury. Never wait to find out if the individual awakens.

Are Head Injuries Common?

Brain damage is frequent. For example, over 700,000 Australians suffer brain injuries, which significantly limit their ability to carry out daily tasks, according to the Australian Bureau of Statistics.

Of them, three out of every four are under 65. Up to two of every three people have brain damage prior to turning 25. Men make up 75% of those who suffer from brain injuries.

Injury to the head is most prevalent in those 75 years of age and older and in those aged 15 to 24. All age groups, however, are susceptible to brain injuries. Numerous incidents, such as auto accidents, falls, being hit by an instrument, and shaken child syndrome, can result in head injuries.

A brain injury can cause moderate symptoms like a headache or serious symptoms like loss of consciousness. Even if symptoms appear mild, it's crucial to get medical help right away if you or someone you know has had a blow to the head or any other kind of brain injury.

First Aid for Head Injury

It's critical to understand how to administer first aid appropriately in the event that you or someone you're with has a head injury. This can increase the likelihood of a full recovery and lessen the probability of additional injuries.

First, use a clean towel to apply direct pressure to the wound if the person is bleeding. Avoid attempting to remove any items that could be embedded in the incision if the bleeding is excessive.

Secondly, carefully apply an ice pack to the affected region for 15 minutes at a time if the patient has a bump or bruise on their head but is not bleeding. Repeat as needed to relieve discomfort.

Thirdly, watch for any indications that the patient's symptoms—such as headache, nausea, vomiting, disorientation, or confusion—are getting worse. If these appear, try to get medical help.

Lastly, do Rescue Breathing if the person is unconscious and not breathing regularly. Next step would be to be recovered in a medical facility, if available in your scenario.

You can guarantee that someone with a brain injury gets the right care and attention by adhering to these guidelines.

Is Throwing Up a Sign of a Brain Injury?

In the event of a head injury, it's critical to watch out for internal bleeding symptoms. If the patient throws up blood, this might be one sign of internal bleeding. The person may also feel queasy or throw up if they have a concussion.

It's common knowledge that youngsters may vomit once due to shock, but if they do so again or more, it means there could be an injury.

Is It OK to Nod Off Following a Head Injury?

One of the most crucial things you can do to prevent brain injuries is to be awake and aware. It might be challenging to accomplish this, particularly if you're feeling queasy or in pain. If you feel like you are going to fall asleep, it is important to resist the temptation and get yourself checked out.

Work-Related Head Injury

Following a head injury, it's important to remain awake for a few reasons. First of all, if you doze off, you won't be able to keep an eye on your symptoms or determine whether they're growing worse. With small toddlers who would typically snooze throughout the day, this might be more difficult.

Maintaining the proper alignment of your spine is crucial if you have any other ailments, such as a neck injury. Sleeping might induce movement, which could exacerbate the condition.

How to Stop a Head Wound from Bleeding

You must get medical help as quickly as possible if you are bleeding from a head injury. You can still perform a few actions to halt the bleeding until assistance comes.

Use a clean cloth or sanitary towel to apply pressure to the wound if the bleeding is the result of a cut or laceration. Don't take off the cloth if it starts to get wet with blood; instead, keep applying pressure, add extra layers of cloth on top if needed.

Head Injury Evaluation

It is not advisable to attempt to seal the wound or reposition the bone if the bleeding originates from an open wound or protrusion of the skin. All you have to do is apply pressure to stop the bleeding.

Never remove an item that is stuck in a wound since doing so might exacerbate the injury. Once more, apply pressure to stop the bleeding.

Typical Reasons for Brain Injuries

Falling is among the most frequent causes of brain injuries. While it can happen at any age, little children and elderly persons are the most likely to experience it. In addition, maltreatment, sports injuries, and auto accidents can result in head traumas.

Other typical reasons for brain injuries consist of:
- Being struck in the head by anything
- Having a head collision with another person or object
- Being in a blast wave during an explosion

When to Consult a Specialist for a Head Injury

We are considering a TEOTWAWKI scenario, but sometimes, for these kind of injuries it is critical that you visit a doctor as soon as possible. This is due to the fact that brain injuries can be hazardous and, if improperly treated, can result in long-term issues.

The following symptoms should prompt you to consult a specialist right away:
- intense headache that won't go away;
- lightheadedness or a ringing sensation in the ears;
- double or blurry vision, speech impediments, vomiting, nausea, convulsions, or seizures;
- you sense something is off and are concerned.

Which Activities Are Safe for Me To Undertake After a Head Injury?

Following a brain injury, there are a few things you can do to aid in your recovery. Get lots of sleep beforehand. Your body requires time to recover itself; provide it this time by obtaining some rest.

Second, eat a balanced diet and stay hydrated. This will support recovery and help your body perform at its peak. Lastly, stay away from activities like lifting large things or playing contact sports, which can strain your head or neck.

Before you do anything rigorous, give your body the time it needs to recuperate completely.

What Distinguishes a Concussion from a Head Injury?

Because they are essentially the same thing, there isn't much distinction between a concussion and a brain injury. Determining the extent of the damage is crucial in order to ascertain if it is a concussion, a simple bump and bruise, or something more serious.

One kind of brain damage that results from a hit to the head or a quick jolt to the body is a concussion. Numerous symptoms, such as headache, nausea, vomiting, dizziness, blurred vision, and memory and attention issues, can be brought on by concussions.

There are situations where this can be more dangerous than concussions and involve brain damage, internal bleeding, and skull fractures. Head injuries need to be treated medically right away since they can be fatal.

Chapter 10: POISONING

Poisoning is caused by exposure to a harmful substance. This could be the result of breathing in, injecting, ingesting, or using another method. Most poisonings usually happen by mistake. Immediate first aid is very important in a poisoning emergency. A person's life can be saved by the first aid you administer before seeking medical attention.

Points to Take

Every year, poison control facilities in the United States receive reports of millions of poisonings. Many lead to demise.

It is crucial to remember that a substance's safety does not automatically follow from a package's lack of a warning label. If someone suddenly gets sick and there's no obvious cause for it, you should think of poisoning. In addition, poisoning should be taken into account if the victim was discovered next to an automobile, furnace, fire, or poorly ventilated space.

It might take some time for poisoning symptoms to appear. However, DO NOT wait for symptoms to appear if you believe someone has been poisoned.

Reasons

Poisoning-causing items include:

- Carbon monoxide gas (produced by space heaters, gas engines, furnaces, and fires)
- Some foods
- Chemical exposure at work
- Drugs include prescription and over-the-counter medications (such as an overdose of aspirin) and illegal substances like cocaine
- Cleaners and detergents for the home

- Both indoor and outdoor plants (consuming poisonous plants)
- Insecticides
- Paints

Depending on the toxin, symptoms might vary but could include:

- Stomach ache
- Red lips due to cyanosis
- Chest ache
- Perplexity
- Throw up diarrhea
- Breathing problems or breathlessness
- Wooziness
- Dual perception
- Tiredness
- High temperature
- Head Pain
- Heart palpitations
- Sensitivity
- Diminished appetite
- Bladder control loss
- Twitching of muscles
- Dizziness and vomiting
- Tiredness and numbness
- Epilepsy
- Bristles or skin rash
- Unconsciousness (coma)
- Strange breath smell
- Weakness

First Aid

For inhalations and some swallowing poisonings:

Verify and keep an eye on the person's respiration, pulse, and airway. Start CPR and rescue breathing if needed.

Verify if the victim has indeed been poisoned. Not always easy to tell. Some symptoms include breath that smells like chemicals, burns around the lips, breathing problems, vomiting, or an odd scent coming from the individual. Find out what poison it is, if you can.

Unless instructed to do so by poison control or a medical expert, DO NOT force someone to throw up.

Make sure the person's airway is clear if they vomit. Put a handkerchief over your fingers and wipe the neck and mouth. Save the vomit if the person has become ill due to a plant component. It could assist professionals in determining which medication can be taken to help reverse the poisoning.

Provide convulsion first aid if the patient begins experiencing convulsions.

Ensure the person is at ease. Once the patient is moved to their left side, they should stay there until medical assistance arrives or is needed.

Take off the garments and give the skin a water wash if the poison has seeped onto it.

In case of inhalation:

Never try to save someone without first alerting others.

Save the individual from the gas, fumes, or smoke if it is safe to do so. To get rid of the smells, open the doors and windows.

Breathe in deeply several times while taking in the fresh air, and then hold your breath. Cover your mouth and nose with a moist towel.

Certain gases can catch fire; therefore, NEVER use a lighter or match to start one.

Once the victim has been pulled out of harm's way, observe and assess the victim's respiration, pulse, and airway. Start CPR and rescue breathing if needed.

Provide immediate assistance for convulsions or eye damage if necessary.

Make sure the person's airway is clear if they vomit. Put a handkerchief over your fingers and wipe the neck and mouth.

NEVER: Give anything by mouth to someone who is unconscious.

Induce vomiting unless you are told to do so by the Poison Control Center or a doctor. A potent toxin that burns the throat on the way down can also cause harm when it comes back up.

Except if instructed to do so by the Poison Control Center or a medical professional, try neutralizing the poison with vinegar, lemon juice, or any other item.

Any "cure-all" form of antidote can be used.

In the event that you believe someone has been poisoned, wait for symptoms to appear.

When to Speak with a Medical Expert

Once you've performed first aid at home, you might need to visit the emergency facility set up in your scenario by EMP, even if some hours are passed. If possible, bring the container with you to the facility. Testing will be done in the facility. In addition, you could require the following therapies and testing:

- inactive carbon;
- oxygen, a ventilator (breathing machine), and a breathing tube via the mouth (intubation) are examples of airway assistance;
- testing for blood and urine;

- chest x-ray ECG (electrocardiogram, or heart tracing) CT (computerized axial tomography) scan;
- liquids passing via a vein (IV);
- locomotive;
- medications to address symptoms, such as antidotes, if any, to undo the effects of poisoning.

When the situation is very serious

The situation is very serious if the person is:

- drowsy or unresponsive;
- breathing heavily or has stopped breathing;
- very anxious or restless;
- being in seizures.

Recognized to have overdosed on drugs or any other substance, whether on purpose or by accident (in these cases, the poisoning usually entails bigger doses, frequently combined with alcohol).

In the following cases, contact your local poison control center or Poison Help at 800-222-1222 in the United States, even after hours, if the catastrophic situation returns normal:

The patient is symptom-free and stable.

The individual will be sent to a nearby emergency facility.

Prepare a detailed account of the patient's symptoms, age, weight, and any additional drugs they might be taking, along with any information you might have regarding the toxin. Find out how much was consumed and how long the person has been exposed to it. When chatting with the poison control center, try to have the pill bottle, pharmaceutical packet, or other suspicious container close at hand so you can consult its label.

What To Do When You're Seeking Assistance

Do the following until assistance arrives, or they are not available at all:

Consumed poison. Take out whatever is still in the person's mouth. Read the label on any suspected poisoning containers and take the necessary precautions if the suspected poison is a chemical, such as a home cleaner.

Poison on the skin. Put on gloves and take off any contaminated clothes. Rinse the skin in a shower or with a hose for 15 to 20 minutes.

The eye was poisoned. Cool or lukewarm water should be used to gently flush the eye for 20 minutes or until further assistance comes.

Swallowed poison. Move the individual as quickly as you can outside in fresh air.

To avoid choking, move the person's head to the side if they vomit.

If there are no indications of life, such as breathing, movement, or coughing, start CPR.

Get someone to gather medication bottles, labeled packets or containers, and any other information regarding the poison to send to the emergency facility set up in your area.

When an Overdose of Opioids Occurs

If naloxone (Narcan) is available and the patient is in danger of overdosing on opioid painkillers, please give it to them. If a patient is in danger of overdosing, medical professionals are increasingly prescribing Narcan injectables. Family members ought to know how to utilize them.

Caution

Syrup of Ipecac. Don't give syrup or ipecac or do anything to induce vomiting. The American Academy of Pediatrics and the American Association of Poison Control Centers are two expert organizations that no longer support the use of ipecac in children or adults who have consumed drugs or other potentially harmful substances. Its efficacy is not well supported by research, and it frequently has unfavorable side effects.

If you still have outdated ipecac syrup bottles in your house, discard them.

Battery buttons. Little children are especially vulnerable to the little, flat batteries found in watches and other devices, especially the bigger, nickel-sized ones. Severe tissue burns can occur from a battery lodged in the esophagus.

If you think a kid might have swallowed one of these batteries, the only thing you could do in a TEOTWAWKI scenario is get an emergency X-ray done immediately to discover the battery's position, if available in any medical facility set up in the area. It will be necessary to remove the battery if it is within the esophagus. It is generally safe to let it continue through the digestive tract if it has already entered the stomach.

Administered patches. In the event that you suspect a kid might have gotten hold of medicated patches—adhesive devices used for transdermal medication delivery—carefully examine the child's skin and take off any that could be attached. Inspect the roof of the mouth as well since the kid might chew on medicinal patches there and become trapped.

Prevention

Know what toxins exist in and around your house. Take precautions to shield small children from dangerous materials. All home chemicals, medications, cleansers, and cosmetics should be kept out of children's reach or kept in cabinets with childproof locks.

Know the plants in your yard, house, and surrounding area. Make sure your kids are informed as well. Delete any toxic plants. Eat no berries, roots, mushrooms, or wild plants unless you are extremely familiar with them.

Children should be taught the risks associated with drugs that contain toxicity.

Label Every Poison

Even if they are labeled, DO NOT keep home chemicals in food containers. In big enough quantities, the majority of nonfood chemicals are toxic.

Report your concerns to the state or federal Environmental Protection Agency or the local health department if you are worried that industrial chemicals could contaminate the land or water in the area. Better to do this now in a normal situation, than in a TEOTWAWKI scenario.

Certain toxins and environmental exposures can induce symptoms and harm even in the absence of significant dosages or physical contact. Thus, in order to prevent major injury, it is crucial to receive treatment as soon as possible. The kind of toxin the individual was exposed to, and the care they received to address the exposure will determine the result.

Chapter 11: FROSTBITE

When skin and underlying tissue freeze as a result of exposure to extremely low temperatures, frostbite develops. In minor cases, frostnip can be self-treated with appropriate first aid, causing redness and numbness; however, more severe stages of frostbite necessitate immediate medical intervention. Treatments for frostbite involve carefully regulated rewarming as well as other treatments such as IV fluids and medicines.

Treating frostbite correctly and quickly is crucial to avoiding consequences, such as irreversible damage. Here's what you should do to properly manage your issue.

Handling Frostbite

The mildest type of cold-related skin damage is frostnip. Frostnip symptoms include:

- redness or paleness of skin;
- minimal discomfort;
- tingling or numbness in cold-exposed bodily areas.

While frostbite might not require a visit from an expert, it is a sign that the skin has begun to get harmed and that further exposure can result in a more serious type of frostbite.

Frostnip can be treated by staying warm. This comprises:

- Reaching a cozy haven
- Wearing layers of dry garments to cover
- Warm air from your lips should be exhaled around the afflicted region with your hands clasped.
- Use body heat to warm the extremity—for example, by placing your fingers in your armpit—

Treating Frostbite

Sometimes, frostbite mimics a burn injury.

Frostbite of the second degree, or superficial, affects the epidermis. Symptoms include:

- Waxy, white skin
- Absence of feeling
- Blossoming blisters with transparent liquid
- If left untreated, second-degree frostbite has the potential to worsen

In the beginning, symptoms of third-degree (deep-tissue) frostbite can resemble those of second-degree frostbite:

- Blisters that turn dark and bleed as the skin thaws
- Turning dark skin
- Loss of tissue

Get Medical Help Right Away if Available

Whenever you suspect frostbite, you should see a doctor right away, in a medical facility. If you are unable to go to it immediately, begin treating the frostbite with basic aid.

In the facility, even after hours from the accident, prompt and expert medical assessment and management of frostbite are essential, as it can be challenging to determine the extent of tissue damage.

The medical staff of the facility will:

- Warm the part that was frostbitten
- Wrap it to shield the skin
- Give painkillers
- Assess to ascertain the severity of the harm

Thrombolytic treatment may be utilized to disintegrate blood clots in third-degree instances in an effort to lower the risk of amputation due to significant tissue damage.

It could take weeks to notice the full degree of tissue damage, so you might need to schedule follow-up sessions to keep an eye on the affected region.

First Aid for Frostbite

If you are unable to travel to a facility immediately, then you should only attempt to treat frostbite.

If there's a chance that the frostbitten skin might freeze again, don't try to defrost it. If the tissue is allowed to stay frozen for a longer period, it will sustain worse damage.

Avoid walking on frostbitten feet unless it's essential to reach a safe place. Stepping on icy feet might exacerbate the tissue damage.

To begin administering first aid, submerge the injured area of the body in warm water (98 to 105 degrees Fahrenheit, or slightly warmer than normal body temperature). Use an unaffected hand to feel the water to make sure it's comfortable and won't burn you if you don't have a thermometer.

Give the frozen region a half-hour soak. Continue to refresh the water in the container as it cools to keep it at a consistent temperature. To help get warm, gently wrap the region with a cloth or a blanket if you don't have access to water.

Warming the skin can cause excruciating agony when the numbness goes away, depending on the extent of the injury. If accessible, you can treat symptoms with an over-the-counter (OTC) non-steroidal anti-inflammatory medication, such as ibuprofen, until you can visit a medical facility.

The skin may begin to blister while it warms up. Please do not pop any of the blisters to prevent infection. After the area has dried, you can put a thick, sterile dressing on it. Verify that the bandages are neither too tight or too loose.

Chapter 12: BURNS AND SCALDS

Let's return to the topic of burns for a moment to also talk about scalds. Scalds and burns are damage to the skin caused by heat. They can both be treated the same way. Dry heat from an iron or fire, for example, is what causes a burn. Something moist, like steam or hot water, causes a scald.

Burns may cause a great deal of discomfort and may also cause:

- peeling or red skin;
- swelling;
- blisters;
- charred or white skin.

It's not always the case that the burn's severity correlates with your discomfort level. A severe burn can be comparatively painless.

Treating Burns and Scalds

Here are some first-aid tips to treat a burn:

Remove the victim from the heat source immediately to stop the burning.

Use cool or lukewarm running water to soothe the burn for twenty minutes. Avoid ice, creams, iced water, or oily substances like butter.

Take off any jewelry or clothing close to the burned region of the skin, including baby diapers; however, leave anything that is adhered to the skin alone.

Use a blanket, for example, to keep the individual warm, but be careful not to rub it against the burned area.

Apply a layer of cling film on the burn to cover it. If you have burns on your hand, you might also use a clean plastic bag.

Treat any discomfort with analgesics such ibuprofen or paracetamol.

If the face or eyes are burned, try to sit up as much as possible; this will help minimize swelling.

When to Seek Medical Assistance if available

Depending on its severity, the possibility of treating a burn at home exists. For small burns, avoid popping any blisters that may form and wipe up the burn.

Serious burns need to be treated by a medical specialist in a facility set up in the scenario. You should visit it ASAP (or as soon as it has been set up) for:

- every burn from chemicals and electricity;
- burns that are severe or large - any burn larger than your hand;
- burns of any size that result in scorched or white skin;
- burns that result in blisters on the face, feet, legs, hands, arms, or genitalia.

One should also get medical help if they have inhaled smoke or fumes. Some symptoms, which might manifest later, include:

- sore throat;
- coughing;
- having trouble breathing;
- face burns.

Following a burn or scald, people who are more vulnerable to the consequences of the burn, such as young children and expectant mothers, should also seek medical assistance.

Before applying a bandage, the afflicted area will be cleansed, and the size and depth of the burn will be evaluated. Skin grafting surgery could be suggested in extreme circumstances.

Types of Burn

How severely your skin is harmed and which layers are impacted are considered when evaluating burns. Skin is composed of three layers:

- The skin's outermost layer, or epidermis
- The layer of tissue just underneath, known as the dermis, is home to hair follicles, nerve endings, sweat glands, and blood vessels.
- The deeper layer of fat and tissue is called subcutaneous fat or subcutis

There exist four primary categories of burns, each characterized by a distinct look and set of symptoms:

- Superficial epidermal burn - When you have this, your skin becomes red, painful, and somewhat swollen, but it does not blister.
- Superficial dermal burn - damages the epidermis and a portion of the dermis; the affected area may appear light pink, hurt, and have tiny blisters.
- Partial thickness burn or deep dermal - Where the epidermis and dermis are injured, a deep dermal or partial thickness burn causes your skin to become red and blotchy. It can also cause your skin to become swollen and blisters, which can either be extremely painful or harmless.
- Full thickness burn – a condition in which the dermis, epidermis, and subcutis are all damaged; the skin is frequently burned away, revealing blackened or pale tissue beneath; the remaining skin is dry, black, white, or brown, free of blisters, and may have a leathery or waxy texture.

Avoiding Scalds and Burns

A lot of newborns and young toddlers have serious burns and scalds. You can take the following actions, for example, to lessen the chance that your kid will experience a major accident at home:

Use your elbow to check the water's temperature before putting your infant or toddler in the bath.

Chapter 13: HEART ATTACK

A heart attack is a medical emergency. If you believe you or someone else is experiencing a heart attack, try to intervene asap. In a normal situation, when experiencing heart attack symptoms, the typical person waits three hours for medical attention. Before they get to a hospital, many heart attack victims pass away. The likelihood of survival increases with the time spent in the emergency room. Timely medical intervention minimizes cardiac damage.

What to do if you suspect someone is suffering a heart attack is covered in this section.

You feel a tight band of pain around your chest. From your chest, the agony radiates to your arms, shoulders, and neck. What could your pain mean? Could it be the big one, or just another heart attack? A disruption in the blood flow to a portion of the heart can result in heart attacks. Heart cells perish, and your heart becomes oxygen-starved if the blood flow is obstructed. Your coronary artery walls may accumulate plaque, a hard substance. Other cells and cholesterol make up this plaque. The rupture of one of these plaques or plaque accumulation might result in a heart attack. The reason why heart attacks happen at certain times is unknown.

A heart attack can occur when you're sleeping or at rest, after a rapid surge in physical activity, outside in the cold, or following an abrupt, severe physical or mental stressor, such as a medical condition. Right, so how is a heart attack handled?

In a normal situation. when you visit the hospital for a possible heart attack, a stethoscope-wielding doctor or nurse will listen to your chest. You'll get a blood test to check for cardiac issues. Your doctor can determine how well your heart is pumping blood using a coronary angiography test. If blood flows through our coronary arteries slowly or not, you have either a blocked or narrowed coronary artery. Additional tests might examine your heart's chambers and valves and look for irregular cardiac rhythms. Doctors can perform an emergency surgery known as angioplasty if you have suffered a heart attack. Blocked or narrowed blood vessels can be opened by this surgery or treatment. Typically, a stent—a tiny, metal mesh tube—is inserted into your artery to help keep it open. Medication to disintegrate the clot in your artery could also be administered. Surgeons may occasionally perform heart bypass surgery to restore blood flow to your heart muscle. Following hospital treatment for a heart attack, you might need to take medication to lower your cholesterol, thin your blood, or protect your heart. You might need to take these medications for the rest of your life. Most heart attack survivors also require cardiac rehabilitation. This will teach you how to live a healthy lifestyle and help you gradually improve your level of activity. After the first attack, your chances of having another heart attack increase. The extent of the damage to your heart, its location, and the precautions you take to avoid another one will determine how well you recover after a heart attack. If your heart cannot pump blood to your body as well as it once did, your heart may suffer heart failure and require lifetime care. After a heart attack, most people may gradually resume their regular activities, but you must take precautions to prevent having another one.

In a TEOTWAWKI scenario all you can do is CPR, until a medical facility is set up in your scenario.

Causes

A heart attack happens when the blood flow that supplies oxygen to the heart is cut off. When the heart muscle runs out of oxygen, it starts to fail.

Symptoms

A heart attack's symptoms might differ from person to person. They might be minor or serious. Subtle or uncommon symptoms are common in women, seniors, and diabetics.

In adults, symptoms might include:

- Alterations in mental health, particularly in older adults;
- Chest discomfort that feels like squeezing, pressure, or fullness. The middle of the chest is where the discomfort usually occurs. It may also be felt in the arms, back, jaw, shoulder, and stomach. It may last for many minutes, or it may come and go;
- Lightheadedness;
- Cold sweat;
- Nausea (more common in women);
- Vomiting;
- Indigestion;
- Arm numbness, pain, or tingling (typically the left arm; however, the right arm may also be impacted or affected alone);
- Respiration difficulty;
- Weakness or exhaustion, particularly in women and elderly persons.

First Aid

If you believe a person is experiencing a heart attack:

- Offer them a seat so they can relax and try not to panic
- Take off any tight apparel
- Find out whether the person takes any medication for chest discomfort, such as nitroglycerin for a known cardiac issue, and help them take it
- Pay attention if the pain does not subside quickly with rest or within three minutes after taking nitroglycerin
- Prepare to give CPR and look for other people to help you if the person is unresponsive, not breathing, unconscious, and has no pulse
- Give CPR for one minute to a kid or newborn who is not breathing, unconscious, unresponsive, and not showing a pulse.

- When using an automated external defibrillator (AED) on someone unconscious and unresponsive without a pulse, follow the directions on the AED

Do Not

Except in cases where assistance is necessary, DO NOT leave the individual alone.

Allowing them to downplay the symptoms and persuade you not to dial for emergency assistance is unacceptable.

AVOID waiting to observe if the symptoms subside.

Until a prescription for a cardiac medication (such as nitroglycerin) has been issued, DO NOT give the patient anything by mouth.

Prevention

Adults should take measures to reduce their risk of heart disease when possible.

Give up smoking. A smoker's risk of heart disease is more than doubled.

Pay close attention to your cholesterol, blood pressure, and diabetes, and do what your doctor suggests.

If you're overweight or obese, lose weight.

Engage in regular exercise to strengthen your heart. Consult your physician before beginning a new exercise regimen.

Eat a heart-healthy diet. Cut back on sweets, red meat, and saturated fats. Consume more poultry, seafood, fresh produce, whole grains, and fruits. You can work with your provider to customize a diet that meets your needs.

Keep your alcohol consumption to a minimum. While having one drink per day is linked to a lower risk of heart attacks, having two or more can harm your heart and lead to other health issues.

Chapter 14: DIABETES

People with glucose intolerance are often prescribed many drugs, devices, and equipment, making first aid for diabetic emergencies a valuable resource. Diabetics must understand how to manage both high and low blood sugar levels.

What is a Diabetic Emergency?

Diabetes is a degenerative disease that impairs the body's ability to make or utilize insulin. One of the body's most significant hormones, insulin, helps control blood sugar levels by giving cells the glucose they need to operate.

Diabetes comes in two varieties:

Type-1 (dependent on external insulin)

Type-2 (not dependent on external insulin)

A diabetic emergency is when the body experiences fluctuations in sugar levels, either too low or too high. These are very serious conditions that need to be treated with diabetic first aid and hospitalization in more severe cases.

Types and Causes of Diabetic Emergency

As noted, the body cannot properly regulate blood sugar levels in people with Type 1 and Type 2 diabetes. In Type 1 diabetes, the immune system attacks and kills insulin-producing cells; in Type 2 diabetes, the body becomes less able to utilize the generated insulin.

Variations in blood sugar levels can lead to a diabetic emergency, but consequences from the disease can also occasionally result in an emergency. The following are typical scenarios in which a person with diabetes needs first aid:

Hypoglycemia

When blood sugar levels fall below the usual range, hypoglycemia sets in. The condition is usually identified as hypoglycemia when the blood sugar falls below 70 mg/dL.

Hypoglycemia can be fatal if left untreated and can result in seizures. However, diabetes can be managed as a temporary ailment if the patient recognizes the symptoms before the condition worsens.

While hypoglycemia can strike at any moment, using insulin or other diabetic treatments often sets it off.

The following situations can cause blood sugar levels to drop below normal:

- When someone administers more insulin than is necessary
- Excessive alcohol intake
- Delays or misses the meal
- High level of physical exertion
- Hyperglycemia

In the same way that too little insulin may result in hyperglycemia, too much insulin may cause hypoglycemia. Sugar levels in this condition stay above normal and may worsen if treatment is not received. In severe situations, hyperglycemia can put a person into a diabetic coma or render them unconscious. For this reason, receiving first aid for diabetes is crucial to improving your health.

Signs to Use First Aid for Diabetes

If you believe you are having a diabetic emergency or witness someone close to you suffering from one, here are some indicators to watch out for to determine the sort of emergency you may be facing:

- Low blood sugar
- Nausea, dizziness, and confusion
- Hunger
- Anxious, Irritable, and shaky
- Rapid pulse and heartbeat
- Sweating, chills, and pale skin
- Tiredness and Weakness
- Headaches
- Seizures
- Weight loss in long-term hypoglycemia
- Loss of consciousness or Coma
- Hyperglycemia
- Tingling sensation in the mouth
- Dizziness or drowsiness, eventually causing unresponsiveness
- Rapid breathing and pulse
- Fruity and sweet breath
- Dry and warm skin
- Excessive thirst

Things to Do in the Event of a Diabetic Emergency

It's critical that you take the following actions if you or someone close to you notices the signs mentioned above.

Hypoglycemia

- Take a seat in a shady spot.

- Give them a sugar-filled meal or beverage. By doing this, the sugar level will be able to return to normal. It might be candies, fizzy drinks, fruit juice, or three tablespoons of sugar.
- Call for medical assistance if your situation doesn't improve.

Hyperglycemia

- Check your heart rate and pulse.

What to Include in Your Diabetes First Aid Kit

First aid kits can help you prepare for emergencies and avoid major consequences if you have them at home. The following items should be kept in the kit you made for yourself:

Hypoglycemia First Aid Kit

- Glucometer with additional strips and a lancet
- Fast-acting glucose, such as vitamins or energy drinks
- Current Prescription List
- ID card for medical purposes (if medical facility is activated in your scenario)
- Extra injection needles

Hyperglycemia First Aid Kit

- A lancet device and Glucose Meter with extra strips
- Extra injection needles
- Even if you need to have everything on hand, it's crucial to check if you have the following things:
- An extra glucometer
- Extra syringes, strips, and lancet devices
- Current Prescription List

Chapter 15: ASTHMA

Asthma is defined as a chronic disease condition in which there is inflammation and constriction of the bronchi, which is responsible for coughing, difficulty breathing, overproduction of mucus, and choking sensation. An asthma episode can become an emergency requiring immediate medical intervention and first aid.

Asthma First Aid Steps

To provide first aid for asthma, use a blue or grey relief puffer:

Step 1: Sit the person upright

Remain cool and comforting.

Don't let them be left alone.

Step 2: Use the blue/grey reliever puffer four times.

Shake the puffer.

Put 1 puff into the spacer.

Ensure that the person takes four breaths from the spacer.

Repeat until they've taken four puffs. If you don't have a spacer, give them one puff as they take one calm, deep inhale and hold it for as long as it feels comfortable. Continue until every puff is taken.

Recall: Shake, one puff, four breaths.

Step 3: Wait four minutes

Give 4 additional puffs of the blue/grey reliever, just like in Step 2, if there is no improvement.

Step 4: Until situation doesn't calm down, continue giving the patient four separate puffs every four minutes, taking four breaths for each puff.

Asthma Flare-Up or Attack

An asthma attack or flare-up worsens lung function and asthma symptoms compared to what you'd usually experience daily. An asthma flare-up can develop extremely fast (in minutes) or slowly (over weeks, days, or hours).

An asthma attack is sometimes referred to as a sudden or severe flare-up of asthma. Asthma emergencies can develop out of an asthma attack very fast, but they can be avoided with prompt care.

If you or a family member suffers from asthma, ensure you have an up-to-date asthma action plan from your doctor and are familiar with the four stages of asthma first aid.

Your physician will:

- give the appropriate prescription;
- assist you in creating a strategy to control your asthma;
- provide you with advice on how to handle your asthma and what to do if your asthma flares up.

If you have symptoms of an asthma attack, stick to your asthma action plan.

Indications That You Require First Aid for Asthma

Asthma action plan should be followed if any of the following symptoms are present. Start asthma first aid if you don't have an asthma action plan or are helping someone with an asthma attack. Avoid waiting till your asthma becomes worse.

Signs of mild to moderate asthma (start asthma first aid):

- little breathing difficulties;
- able to talk in full sentences;
- capable of moving or walking;
- may have a wheeze or cough.

Severe asthma symptoms (start asthma first aid and search for help):

- evident breathing difficulties;
- can't pronounce a complete phrase in a single breath;
- pulling the skin around the base of the neck or in between the ribs;
- may have wheeze or cough;
- the duration of the painkiller is shorter than normal.

Signs of life-threatening asthma (start providing first aid and help as much as possible):

- breathing difficulties (gasping for air);
- only able to utter one or two words in a breath;
- perplexed or worn out;
- lips are turning blue;
- symptoms are rapidly becoming worse;
- collapsing;
- using a reliever inhaler and experiencing little to no relief;

- may no longer have a cough or wheeze.

During asthma crises, stick to your action plan.

Learn the first four stages of asthma first aid.

Everyone must be aware of the four asthma first aid stages.

Salbutamol, sometimes known as your "blue puffer," is a common reliever medication. These are available over the counter from a chemist.

It is safe to use blue reliever medicine even if you are unsure whether or not the person is experiencing an asthma attack.

The situation become very critic if:
- the individual isn't breathing;
- their asthma worsens or stays the same abruptly;
- no asthma medicine is on hand, and the person is suffering an attack;
- the individual isn't sure if they have asthma;
- the individual has been diagnosed with anaphylaxis, even if no skin symptoms exist, an adrenaline autoinjector should be administered before pain relievers.

Additional First Aid Guidelines for Asthma

When it comes to asthma, not everyone takes the same medicine.

Bricanyl (terbutaline), another blue reliever, is used by certain persons. It is available in a special type of inhaler called a Turbuhaler.

Others use "dual-purpose" relievers. Budesonide and formoterol are combined as a dual-purpose reliever, taken "as needed."

When used as needed, the dual-purpose reliever's budesonide and formoterol combination soothes symptoms and reduces the chance of severe asthma flare-ups. It accomplishes this by reducing airway inflammation and releasing constricted airway muscles.

Note: these medications may also be provided to you as a "preventer." Regarding what to use during an asthma attack or flare-up, always heed your doctor's directions on your asthma action plan.

Some patients could use the same medication as a preventive measure and a relief.

Asthma symptoms in a severe allergic reaction (anaphylaxis)

Similar asthma symptoms can also occur in those experiencing anaphylaxis, a severe allergic reaction. Follow the instructions on any anaphylaxis action plan that the person may have.

Suppose someone with a documented allergy to food, insects, or medications experiences acute breathing difficulties (such as wheezing, a persistent cough, or a hoarse voice), even without skin symptoms. In that case, they should get an adrenaline injector first, followed by an asthma reliever.

Thunderstorm Asthma

When a certain kind of thunderstorm and large levels of grass pollen in the air come together during grass pollen season, people who suffer hay fever or asthma may have severe symptoms.

Chapter 16: BLEEDING

Discover the most important first aid procedures and how to stop serious bleeding in emergencies. First, try applying direct pressure to stop the bleeding. After the bleeding has stopped, securely wrap the incision with a cloth, gauze, or towel without stopping blood flow.

If it is severe bleeding and will not stop with direct pressure, build a tourniquet, a tight band that limits blood flow to prevent the patient from entering shock.

Your emergency first aid pack should have the following items: gauze, aspirin, bandages, one emergency blanket, two pairs of non-latex gloves, two triangle bandages, and tweezers.

How to Provide First Aid to Stop Bleeding

Most people's initial reaction in an emergency is to find out how to get on the phone and dial 911 as quickly as possible. Though it's a valuable instinct you should never disregard, are you equipped to treat an injured person or yourself in a TEOTWAWKI scenario?

Everyone should be familiar with the fundamentals of first aid so they can take care of themselves or other injured parties in an emergency. If you're fortunate enough to summon an ambulance that will arrive in minutes, every moment matters in an emergency. Stopping serious bleeding before expert medical care comes may make a big difference in a person's recovery, and in certain cases, it may even save their life.

Things To Do Before Helping a Wounded Person

Being able to assist someone in an emergency requires first being able to identify someone who needs assistance in the first place. A person who is bleeding may not always scream for assistance, and the adrenaline of the situation may make it harder for them to perceive pain or realize how serious their injury is.

In an emergency, pay attention to anyone nearby who could be in need, even if you are unharmed. Ensure your safety before trying to help them; if you are a victim, you cannot assist anybody. If the wounded person is on a hill, attempt to gently assist them or carry them up to a sidewalk; if they are in the middle of a crowd, move them to a clear area. Ideally, you should transport the injured person to a safe, level surface.

Try to expose the bleeding wound before tending to someone's injuries, especially if you are unsure of the source of the bleeding. Never try to extract anything from the wound or push anything that is trapped or difficult to remove.

Applying Direct Pressure

Using a large gauze pad, shirt, towel, or other folded fabric to direct pressure to the injured area is one of the most crucial methods for quickly stopping serious bleeding. Don't remove the first cloth or release any pressure if the blood seeps through it; instead, get another cloth to lay over it. Replace the cloth every ten minutes or until help arrives, depending on when the bleeding stops.

Once the bleeding seems to have stopped, use any resources on hand to securely tie the cloth in place (e.g., neckties, shoelaces, pieces of sheet, etc.). Tighten the knot "as tight as it takes" to prevent the wound from actively bleeding; otherwise, you run the danger of severing the limb's blood supply and defeating the purpose of the tourniquet.

If the person is bleeding profusely from their arm or leg, keep the limb above the level of their heart.

How to Use Tourniquets to Stop Serious Bleeding

A tourniquet is a tight bandage to halt blood flow to a wound and prevent shock in the affected patient.

Generally speaking, there are two circumstances in which a tourniquet should be applied:

- If elevation and direct pressure are administered at the same time, and the bleeding doesn't appear to be stopped or slowing down
- If maintaining direct pressure is impossible

Only in cases of extreme uncontrollable bleeding, after all other options have been exhausted, should a tourniquet be used. This technique is frequently required for people in dire situations, including auto accidents, serious cuts, gunshot wounds, or crushed limbs. Although a first responder should apply a tourniquet, you can learn how to do it independently if you need to use one before medical assistance comes.

According to Very Well Health, homemade tourniquets can be effective up to 30 to 35 percent of the time. Remember that tourniquets are only meant to be applied to wounds on the limbs; they cannot be used on wounds on the head, neck, or chest. Remember that a tourniquet should only be used following the application of direct pressure and only when the bleeding cannot be stopped or slowed down by direct pressure alone.

To assemble a tourniquet utilizing supplies you already have at home, you'll need something to wrap around the limb, such as a belt, towel, triangular bandage, or shirt.

You'll also need something to serve as a "windlass," such as a stick, spoon, or pencil. The windlass is a lever used to tighten the tourniquet.

Initially, identify the bleeding source. While placing a tourniquet can be extremely unpleasant for the injured individual, it is frequently an essential step that could save their life or a limb.

Once done, place the tourniquet object a few inches above the wound. The area of the limb nearest the heart is where the tourniquet should be placed. The tourniquet must be placed above the joint if the damage is below the elbow or knee. Don't forget to allow enough length when you tie the fabric into a knot.

Tie the loose ends of the tourniquet (fabric) around your stick (or any other object you use as a windlass), lay it on the knot, and twist the stick to apply more pressure. Keep turning the stick until the bleeding has stopped or has greatly decreased.

Remember that a tourniquet should not be used for more than two hours. To help in case of further medical aid, you should write down the time you applied the tourniquet.

What Equipment Should I Include in My Quick Emergency First Aid Kit?

Even though you might not always have access to an emergency first aid kit, it's a good idea to assemble a kit with the necessities and keep it in your house and car. Some items you should always have on hand for your kit include (but are not restricted to):

- Gauze
- Tweezers
- Aspirin
- Bandages (assorted sizes)
- 1 emergency blanket
- Gauze roller bandage
- 2 pairs of nonlatex gloves
- 2 triangular bandages

Chapter 17: STROKE

During a stroke, timing is critical. A stroke may result in losing awareness or balance, increasing the risk of falling. The following actions should be taken if you suspect that you or someone around is experiencing a stroke:

- As you tend to someone else experiencing a stroke, ensure they are positioned securely and comfortably. They should be supported if they throw up and rest on one side with their head slightly lifted
- Check to see if they are breathing. Do CPR if they are not breathing. If they have trouble breathing, loosen any restrictive clothes, such as a scarf or tie
- Speak in a soothing, collected tone
- To keep them warm, cover them with a blanket
- Don't offer them any food or liquids
- Do not move the person if they exhibit any weakness in a limb
- Keep a close eye on the person to see whether their condition changes. Be ready to describe symptoms and when they first appeared in case of further medical aid. Be careful to indicate if the victim hit their head or fell

Know the Signs of a Stroke

The degree of the stroke will determine how severe the symptoms are. You must be aware of any dangers before you can help. The FAST acronym can be used to check for warning symptoms for stroke.

FAST stands for:

- **Face**: Does one side of the face droop, or is it numb?
- **Arms**: Is one arm weaker or number than the other? When attempting to elevate both arms, does one arm remain lower than the other?
- **Speech**: Is the speech garbled or slurred?
- **Time**: It is necessary to request help immediately if any of the preceding questions apply to you.

Additional signs of a stroke include:

- impaired, hazy, or absent vision, particularly in one eye;
- feeling numb, weak, or tingling on one side of the body;
- nausea;
- bowel control or loss of bladder;
- migraine;
- feeling lightheaded or dizzy;
- consciousness or loss of balance;

Don't wait to see if you or someone else exhibits signs of a stroke. Take symptoms seriously, even if they are mild or subside. The degeneration of brain cells occurs in a matter of minutes. By administering clot-busting medications within 4.5 hours, the American Heart Association (AHA) and American Stroke Association (ASA) recommendations suggest reducing the likelihood of impairment. It is also stated in these recommendations that mechanical clot removals can be carried out as late as 24 hours following the onset of stroke symptoms.

Causes of Stroke

A stroke happens when bleeding or an interruption in the blood flow to the brain.

An ischemic stroke occurs when a blood clot blocks an artery leading to the brain. One of the main causes of ischemic strokes is plaque accumulation in the arteries. A thrombotic stroke occurs when a clot develops inside a brain artery. A cerebral embolic stroke may result from clots that form elsewhere in the body and move to the brain.

A cerebral blood artery breaks and bleeds, resulting in a hemorrhagic stroke.

The signs of a ministroke, or transient ischemic attack (TIA), may be difficult to diagnose. It is a quick event. The symptoms usually disappear in less than 24 hours and don't persist for more than five minutes. A transient obstruction of blood supply to the brain is the cause of transient ischemic attacks (TIAs). It indicates that a more serious stroke could be on the horizon.

Stroke Recovery

Following treatment and first assistance, the healing phase from a stroke might vary. It relies on several variables, including the patient's medical history and the speed at which they got therapy.

Acute care is the term for the initial phase of recovery. It takes place in a hospital. Your condition is evaluated, stabilized, and treated at this point. A person recovering from a stroke may be hospitalized for as long as seven days. However, the path to recovery is often far from done after that.

After a stroke, rehabilitation is often the next phase of recovery. It may take place in an inpatient rehabilitation center or the hospital.

Rehabilitative objectives are:

- Strengthen motor abilities
- Increase mobility
- To promote movement in the injured limb, minimize using the intact limb
- Apply range-of-motion treatment to relieve tense muscles

Caregiver Information (if the scenario returns to normal)

Your work as a stroke survivor's caregiver may be difficult. However, being prepared and having a support network might make it easier to deal with. You must discuss the reason for the stroke with the hospital's medical staff. You should also talk about potential courses of action for therapy and averting further strokes.

Some of the caring duties you may have while recovering are as follows:

- weighing the choices for recovery;
- scheduling for medical appointments and transportation to rehabilitation;
- weighing the possibilities for assisted living, nursing homes, and adult daycare;
- making plans for in-home medical care;
- overseeing the financial and legal requirements of the stroke victim;
- controlling food requirements and prescriptions;
- modifying the house to increase mobility;

After being discharged from the hospital, a stroke victim could still experience ongoing speech, movement, and cognition issues. They could also be bedridden or restricted to a tiny space. As their caretaker, you might have to assist them with daily activities like eating, talking, and personal hygiene.

Make sure you take care of yourself in all of this. You can't care for your loved one if you're sick or stressed out. When you need assistance, ask friends and family for it, and use routine respite care. Try to obtain a full night's sleep every night and maintain a healthy diet. If you're feeling sad or overwhelmed, exercise regularly and seek assistance from your physician.

Outlook

A stroke survivor's prognosis is difficult to forecast because it relies on various factors. Don't wait to seek emergency assistance as soon as you suspect you may be having a stroke, as the timing of treatment is crucial. Diabetes, blood clots, and heart disease are a few other illnesses that can make stroke recovery more difficult and time-consuming. Participation in rehab is also important for regaining mobility, normal speech, and motor skills. And last, just as with any major illness, recovery will be greatly aided by having a good outlook and a supportive network of loving individuals.

Chapter 18: EPILEPSY SEIZURES

You can protect someone during a seizure by being ready to act quickly. However, you can help in protecting someone from danger during one. Seizures vary in their level of risk, although most are not life-threatening. Preserving their safety should be your primary concern if you wish to help them.

What Seizures Look Like

The most common kind of seizure that comes to mind is the grand mal seizure, sometimes referred to as a generalized tonic-clonic seizure. They are terrifying to watch, and those who have one hardly understand or remember what's happening.

There is a pattern to these seizures:

- It appears that the person "checked out." When you speak with them, they won't respond. You can shake or wave a hand, but they won't respond. They may collapse.
- Their body tenses, making them as stiff as a board. This is the tonic phase. (It lasts for a short while.)
- A succession of jerky motions follow. This is the clonic phase. (It might last several minutes or a few seconds.)
- The jerking eventually ceases, and they become conscious and able to speak again, though they could remain confused or clumsy for a little while.
- A person experiencing a generalized seizure may be dangerous as they cannot defend themselves from injury and are ignorant of their surroundings. The uncontrolled thrashing increases their risk of getting hurt.
- Focal seizures are different. They often last a little over a minute or two and are less intense.

- Part of their body, such as an arm, may become rigid or floppy. Some jerky, rhythmic, or repetitive motions start in one area of the body and extend to other sections. Either zoning out or staring at nothing is possible. They are powerless over what is happening, whether they know it or not. They will have forgotten everything when it's over.

What You Can Do

It all comes down to taking precautions. In the case of a generalized tonic-clonic seizure:

- allow them space;
- clear the area of any sharp or hard objects, such as furniture and glassware;
- cushion their head;
- tighten your clothes over their neck if it's safe to do so;
- avoid trying to restrain them or impede their motions;

Keep everything out of their mouths. It's a common misconception that you may swallow your tongue during a seizure. However, putting something in their mouth risks breaking their teeth or having them bite you. Turn their head to one side if it's not moving.

When the seizure begins, look at your watch to measure how long it lasts. Remember, even though it might seem like an emergency, it is not one.

To help keep their airway open, gently turn them onto their side after the jerking stops.

Move the individual away from dangers like traffic, stairs, and water if they have milder seizures, such as a bit of staring or trembling of the arms or legs.

Never leave a person who has experienced a seizure alone. Remain until they can react appropriately to your questions and are completely aware of their location.

Talk quietly. Should they appear perplexed or afraid, reassure them and explain what they missed. Give them nothing to eat or drink until they have fully healed.

Rescue Medications/Treatments

Certain medications and therapies are appropriate and useful in particular circumstances. Known as "rescue medications," they should only be used in an emergency to help stop a seizure as soon as possible. They should not be used in place of regular prescriptions. These can be given depending on the situation:

Orally - Swallowed in pill form

Nasally - Sprayed up the nose

Buccally - Placed between the cheek and the gum to dissolve

Sublingually - Placed under the tongue to dissolve

Rectally - Administered via a gel through the anus

Benzodiazepines are the most often utilized drugs because of their rapid bloodstream penetration and ability to act on the brain to halt seizures. They include:

Diazepam - given orally (if the individual is awake);

Valtoco - as a nasal spray;

Diastat – rectally;

Lorazepam - sublingual, orally (if the individual is awake);

Midazolam - administered orally, buccally, or by the nose (Nayzilam).

The situation becomes more critical if

- The seizure lasts longer than five minutes.
- It is a child's first seizure.
- Not long after the first seizure, another one starts.
- The individual does not "wake up" after the motions cease.
- The individual was injured during the seizure.

Further aid could be necessary if the patient has any other medical conditions, such as diabetes or heart problems.

Chapter 19: HYPOTHERMIA

When the body temperature drops below 95 °F (35 °C), hypothermia sets in. Any circumstance in which the body loses more heat to the surroundings than it produces might result in hypothermia.

If severe hypothermia is not treated quickly, it can be fatal.

What is Hypothermia?

Many mechanisms in the human body work together to keep the body's core temperature at a steady 98,6 °C. One need only be in an environment colder than their body temperature to be in danger of developing hypothermia—they will still "donate" heat to the atmosphere even in subzero conditions.

A person's temperature will drop if the heat they produce—which they continually do via muscular contractions and metabolic processes—belongs to them less than the heat they lose to the environment.

The four ways the human body loses heat are as follows:

Conduction: the direct transmission of body heat to an item that is colder than the body (laying on a cold surface, for instance, will conduct body heat away from the body and onto the surface).

Convection: The process through which heat is removed from the skin by moving air or liquid (wind and water colder than body temperature, for example, promote heat loss).

Radiation: Heat is dispersed into the surrounding environment through radiation resulting from electromagnetic waves. For instance, if the air temperature is lower than the body's, heat will escape through exposed skin, and children are especially susceptible to this.

Evaporation: Heat is removed from the skin by evaporation, which converts fluid on the skin into vapor. People with damp skin, such as those who are clammy or have burns, may lose heat more quickly.

Medical conditions can occasionally result in hypothermia. For instance, a person suffering a stroke or a diabetic enduring a hypoglycemic episode may find herself lying immobilized for a while, unable to fend against the cold.

There are two natural reactions to becoming cold, including:

Behavioral: A person with this behavior will try to move around to create heat and look for shelter to prevent more heat loss.

Physiological: to stay warm, the body diverts blood to the core; goose bumps are caused by hair standing on end trapping warm air around the body; we shudder to generate more heat; and hormones are released by the body to increase metabolism.

If these measures are ineffective, hypothermia will take place.

Hypothermia Symptoms

There are three phases of hypothermia: mild, moderate, and severe. The temperature ranges of the various phases can classify the indications and symptoms of hypothermia:

Signs and symptoms of moderate hypothermia (95 °F to 89 °F, 35 °C to 32 °C) include:

- cool and pale to the touch as blood vessels constrict in the skin;
- drowsiness, lethargy, or sluggish responses;
- numbness in the extremities;
- shivering;

- elevated respiration and heart rate.

Signs and symptoms of mild hypothermia (89°F to 82 °F, 32 °C to 28 °C) include:

- lowering the level of consciousness;
- urine incontinence brought on by the kidneys' increased workload from moving blood to the main organs;
- stopped shivering;
- slower breathing, blood pressure, and heart rates.

Signs and symptoms of severe hypothermia (below 82 °F - 28 °C) include:

- unconscious and unable to respond;
- if someone becomes too cold, their heart beats more slowly and irregularly and eventually stops;
- lack of reaction to light in the pupil of the eye;
- stiff muscles, which might make one feel as though they are in rigor mortis;
- respiratory effort and pulses may exist but be difficult to see.

Myth About Hypothermia

One common misconception about hypothermia is that your head loses more heat than any other area of your body. That is untrue. Any skin surface that is exposed to the environment loses heat. The surface area of an adult's head makes up around 10% of their entire body.

With the probable exception of our hands, which combined account for only 4% of our body surface area, the majority of the time, our bodies are covered. As a result, we feel colder in our heads than the rest of our insulated bodies.

A person would lose just as much heat from an exposed head if they were to expose another area of their body, such as their belly, which likewise accounts for 10% of the typical adult body.

There is no particular reason why parents should cover their children's heads to prevent them from becoming cold; rather, this is just common sense. It is more related to how big the head is in relation to the body. Since an infant's head makes up more than 20% of their body surface area after birth, having their head exposed increases heat loss and increases the danger of hypothermia in less time than it would take for an adult.

Potential Causes of Hypothermia

The following are some things that might make someone more vulnerable to hypothermia:

Children – Young children are particularly vulnerable to hypothermia because they lack the self-defense skills necessary to keep warm in a variety of environmental settings. In general, they also lose heat more quickly than adults do. Covering their heads will stop a substantial amount of heat loss because of how big their head is in comparison to their body.

Old age: As skin nerve endings are lost, the capacity of older people to detect temperature changes is compromised. They also produce less heat because they have lower metabolic rates and less fat, both of which have insulating properties. Social considerations also come into play, as older people are more likely to be unwilling to use heating for financial reasons and may be socially isolated, which allows them to live alone and suffer for extended periods without anybody noticing.

Dementia or immobilizing illness – Hypothermia can strike anyone who has dementia or other immobilizing conditions if they are unable to care for themselves on their own, either mentally or physically. Individuals who have dementia may be especially vulnerable if they venture outside in cold weather without first dressing appropriately.

Alcohol and other drugs: Alcohol relaxes blood vessels, increasing blood flow to the skin's surface and giving the illusion of flushed skin and a warm feeling. This is why alcohol makes people feel cozy. Due to the increased rate of heat loss, this also significantly raises the risk of hypothermia for intoxicated individuals who are outside in cold weather. Moreover, it decreases metabolism, which reduces the production of internal heat. Additionally, alcohol inhibits judgment, making it less likely for the user to recognize their physical condition and the surroundings, much alone take precautions to prevent heat loss. Any other substance that alters the mind raises similar concerns.

Water immersion: Individuals will lose a lot of heat if they submerge themselves in water that is cooler than their body temperature for any length of time. Anyone who may have spent a significant amount of time in damp clothing owing to perspiration or incontinence is the other individual who is in danger.

Severe Hypothermia Can Be Fatal

Generally, mild hypothermia (body temperature between 95 °F to 89 °F (35°C and 32°C) is easily treated. But when the body temperature falls below 32°C, the chance of dying rises.

If the core body temperature is less than 82°F (28°C), the situation is potentially fatal. A person at this temperature will be extremely cold to the touch, inflexible, unresponsive, breathing, without a pulse, and with fixed pupils—that is, insensitive to changes in light. They might not be dead, but they will look that way.

First Aid For Severe Hypothermia

These are some first-aid measures for severe hypothermia:

Keep an eye on the person's respiration. If they are suffering from acute hypothermia, they may stop breathing altogether or breathe in a dangerously shallow or slow way.

If the person is not breathing regularly, is unresponsive or unconscious, or is not moving, start Rescue Breathing, or cardiopulmonary resuscitation (CPR) right away if you no longer feel the heartbeat.

Never assume a person is dead. Severe hypothermia can cause a person to breathe just once per minute and have a pulse rate of less than twenty beats per minute. Always assume they are alive.

First Aid for All Cases of Hypothermia

Throughout all phases of hypothermia, the following first aid advice is applicable. Preventing more heat loss is the first thing to do in any incidence of hypothermia. To do this, the four mechanisms of heat loss are eliminated, namely:

Conduction: if at all possible, take the person off of a cold surface. Put them on a warm surface if possible, or at least somewhere dry that won't allow any more heat to escape.

Convection: Take the victim out of a damp or windy area. While providing blankets is a nice idea, the main goal should be to get them into shelter.

Radiation: To prevent radiant heat loss, cover as much of the person as you can. Particularly cover the head of a younger child.

Evaporation: People who are sweaty and damp will lose heat through evaporation. When possible, dry your skin, and take off any damp clothes as soon as you can.

Avoid giving the person a massage or rub, and don't allow them to help you. They run the danger of going into cardiac arrest; therefore, keep them still, especially below 89 °F (32 °C).

If moving them outside is not an option, cover their head, protect them from the wind, and keep their body warm by insulating them from the chilly ground. If the person is severely or moderately hypothermic, move the sufferer as gently as you can. The heart is particularly susceptible below about 87°F (30 °C), and there are case reports of even seemingly insignificant actions such as turning someone over causing a cardiac arrest.

Take off any damp clothes and put on dry, warm clothing in its stead. Cover the person's head.

Instead of submerging the victim in hot water, try to warm them up. Ensure that the people are dry. To keep whatever heat they are creating within, insulate them from the outside world. Warm the individual gradually using any accessible heat source, such as heaters, heat packs, hot water bottles, or an electric blanket. The individual shouldn't be too near to the heat source or too hot. Whatever heat source is used simply has to be warmer than the individual supplying heat; a steady, progressive warming is optimal. Be cautious not to overheat anything that is applied near the skin, such as heat packs or hot water bottles, as this might cause burns or affect the person's sense of skin temperature. To concentrate warmth on the center region, if employing several little heat sources, such as heat packs, place them mostly around the torso, into the armpits, and in the groin. Share body heat: Lay down next to someone and make skin-to-skin contact while taking off your clothes to warm their body. After that, wrap a blanket across both bodies and, if you can, get into a sleeping bag.

Alcohol reduces the body's capacity to retain heat; therefore, avoid giving it. Have the person sip warm, non-alcoholic drinks if they are awake and able to swallow. If they're throwing up, don't give them any liquids.

Remain with the person at all times; don't leave them alone.

Keep an eye on the person's breathing at all times. If you are certified to do CPR, start it right once if the person stops breathing and you no longer feel the heartbeat. Keep performing CPR until the victim begins breathing on their own or further aid arrives.

Never assume the person is dead; CPR can save the life of someone who appears to be dead due to severe hypothermia. They may be cold to the touch, stiff, with frozen pupils, no pulse, and no breathing; nevertheless, they might still be alive.

How to Avoid Hypothermia When You're Outdoors

If you are unprepared, even a brief exposure to cold weather might be dangerous. Shivering and feeling numb or chilly indicate excessive heat loss in the body.

Among the simple ways to prevent hypothermia are:

- Avoid spending too much time outside in the cold.
- Recognize when there are meteorological conditions that might raise the danger of hypothermia and take appropriate action. For instance, seek refuge during a snowstorm.
- Do not rely on the car heater to keep warm when driving in cold weather, especially if there is a danger that ice or snow could accumulate on the road and increase the likelihood of an accident. To increase your chances of avoiding hypothermia in the case of an accident or snowfall, dress appropriately for the cold outside the car and turn down the heat.
- To retain body heat, dress in several layers as opposed to a single, heavy one. Natural fibers like wool are great at holding heat.
- Utilize a weatherproof outer layer to remain dry.
- Use scarves, socks, and gloves, with spares to replace when wet.
- Put on insulated footwear.
- Use a warm head covering.
- Make sure your boots and clothing fit properly. You are more likely to experience hypothermia if your blood circulation is compromised.
- Consume a lot of liquids.
- Eat often.
- Take regular breaks to lower the chance of physical exhaustion.
- Make sure you have a professional thermometer in your first aid box so you can monitor your body temperature precisely.
- Remove your wet clothes as soon as possible.
- Steer clear of coffee, cigarettes, and alcohol.
- Ensure that a sufficient number of waterproof matches are included in your kit.
- Use a buddy system.

- Use the 'buddy system' and keep an eye out for each other's warning signals when engaging in any outdoor activity that has a risk of hypothermia, such as hiking or mountaineering. Mental disorientation may prevent you from identifying your hypothermia symptoms. First aid training is highly recommended.

Hypothermia at home

It is possible to suffer hypothermia at home. Hypothermia is more common in the elderly and in some medically ill individuals. One way to lower the risk is to:

- ensuring that the house has enough heat;
- seeking help from government agencies for help with food, clothing, and heating if necessary;
- undergoing routine medical checkups.

Chapter 20: TICK BITE

While tick bites are often not very harmful, they can occasionally result in an allergic response or other significant sickness. It is not a good idea to brush off, forget, and deal with tick bites later. Certain ticks may harbor microorganisms that lead to illnesses and other issues. After being bitten, the skin may become discolored, and the affected region may swell or hurt.

When it comes to tick bites, prevention and treatment are the most crucial things to consider to avoid health issues.

How to Identify Tick Bites

The paralysis tick, or Ixodes holocyclus, is the most frequent tick species that attacks people in Australia. Once they bite their warm-blooded hosts, these parasites—sometimes called "mean little suckers"—feed on their blood.

Both humans and animals can be harmed by tick bites, which can spread germs and viruses that can lead to a number of illnesses. Some of these illnesses, such as rocky mountain spotted fever, anaplasmosis, tularemia, and Lyme disease, can be extremely dangerous to one's health.

Ticks are a kind of arachnid related to spiders and mites, too. During each step of their life cycle, from the egg that hatches into a larva to the nymph that grows into an adult tick, they change in size and form.

Though there are many different kinds of ticks, one of the most prevalent ones is the paralysis tick.

Signs and Symptoms

Many of the conditions brought on by tick bites have comparable symptoms, including:

- Fever or high body temperature
- Shivers
- Chest discomfort and aches
- Headache
- Tiredness
- Irritation or itching (typically appears later)
- Skin rash

Tick-induced rashes can sometimes be signs of an illness. Bullseye-shaped red dots on the skin might be the first indications of Lyme disease, whereas little reddish or purple spots are frequently linked to Rocky Mountain Spotted Fever.

How Do Tick Bites Look and Feel?

When they bite, ticks do not fully burrow beneath the skin. As they feed, they can bury portions of their heads for up to 10 days inside the skin of a human or an animal.

Most of the time, a person getting bitten won't feel anything. Nonetheless, the bite site may seem somewhat swollen and red.

Seek quick medical attention if you believe that a tick has bitten you or someone else.

First Aid Treatment For Tick Bites

First, take out the tick as soon as possible and with caution.

To remove the tick as near to your skin as possible, use tweezers or fine-tipped forceps. It is important to avoid the tick breaking apart and leaving its mouthparts in the skin; therefore, avoid simply grabbing the body, which may be soft and swollen with blood. Once you get it in your hands, gently but firmly pull out the tick, moving it straight backward from the direction of entry.

When pulling the tick, avoid twisting or squeezing it, and do not try to touch it with your bare hands. Moreover, attempting to remove a tick with petroleum jelly, nail paint, or a hot match is not advised; instead, you need to remove it, not encourage it to let go forcibly.

Take a photo and place it in a container once it has been properly removed. You and your healthcare practitioner can identify the tick's species and assess any potential concerns by taking pictures of it.

Use warm water and soap to wash your hands and the region that was bitten thoroughly. As an alternative, you can clean the bite with an iodine scrub or rubbing alcohol.

When To Get Medical Attention

Seek prompt medical assistance in the event that any of the following symptoms appear:

- Paralysis symptoms, such as tingling, incoordination, and weakness
- Severe pain or migraine
- Chest ache
- Palpitations and an erratic pulse
- Difficulty breathing
- Or any other serious symptoms

There's no need to visit a doctor for most tick bites. On the other hand, if you try to remove a tick and some of it ends up in your skin, it's essential to get medical attention.

If further symptoms appear (paralysis, rash, fever, etc.), you should visit the ER or have them examined for treatment.

Most tick bites are not harmful and don't need to be treated by a doctor. However, some ticks—such as paralysis ticks—can transmit pathogenic bacteria that lead to illnesses like Lyme disease and Rocky Mountain spotted fever.

The public is still at risk for infections like Lyme disease and others spread by ticks. Children and older people are among the many individuals who are most vulnerable to its effects.

The chance of tick bite illnesses in the future can be reduced by understanding proper treatment and prevention.

Chapter 21: SHOCK

The first medical attention provided to someone experiencing shock is known as shock first aid. Shock is a dangerous condition that occurs as a result of insufficient blood flow to the body. Symptoms of shock include rapid heartbeat, low blood pressure, shallow breathing, fatigue, and anxiety.

What Is Shock First Aid Treatment?

Providing first aid to someone who has experienced shock is known as shock first aid treatment. Shock needs to be treated right away. Up to 1 in 5 shock victims pass away as a result of it. More than a million cases of shock are reported to hospital emergency departments in the U.S. annually.

What Is Shock?

Shock is a severe, life-threatening condition that occurs when your body does not get sufficient blood flow.

If there is insufficient blood flow to your organs, they may not receive enough oxygen, which could lead to their failure. In addition, shock can result in hypoxia, or low oxygen levels in the body's tissues, and cardiac arrest.

What Causes Shock?

There are several conditions that may trigger shock, including:

- Low blood volume
- Your heart is not pumping blood well enough
- Certain medications that impair cardiac function
- Excessive dilatation, or widening of your blood vessels
- Your nervous system is being damaged

What Are the Four Main Types of Shock?

There are several types of shock. These include distributive, obstructive, cardiogenic, and hypovolemic shocks.

Hypovolemic Shock

Hypovolemic shock occurs due to low blood volume. A low blood volume indicates that less blood than usual enters your heart with each pulse. Consequently, your body is receiving less blood than usual. Hypovolemic shock might result from:

Excessive bleeding from cuts or other wounds on the outside.

Severe internal bleeding brought on by an ulcer, a blood vessel break, or an ectopic pregnancy—a pregnancy that has burst outside of your uterus.

Other bodily fluid loss as a result of severe burns, pancreatitis, intestinal wall perforation, severe diarrhea, severe vomiting, renal problems, overuse of diuretics (medications that flush the body of water and salt), or untreated diabetes.

Cardiogenic Shock

When your heart gets damaged to the point where it cannot pump as much blood as your body requires, you might experience cardiogenic shock. The following are the most typical causes of cardiogenic shock:

- A myocardial infarction, or heart attack
- An issue with a heart valve
- Irregular heartbeat, or arrhythmia
- Rupture or infection of the heart muscle (myocarditis)
- Tear or inflammation in the heart valve (endocarditis)

Obstructive Shock

An obstruction in your heart, veins, or arteries that stops your blood from flowing normally might cause obstructive shock. An accumulation of fluid in your chest cavity may potentially be the cause. This is a list of causes of obstructive shock:

- Lung clot caused by blood (pulmonary embolism)
- Tension pneumothorax, or trapped air between your lung and chest wall
- Fluid or blood buildup in the space between your outer heart sac (cardiac tamponade) and heart muscle

Distributive Shock

Your blood vessels dilate (widen excessively), which might result in distributive shock. Your blood pressure drops as a result, and your organs don't get enough oxygen and blood flow. Different kinds of distributive shock exist.

These consist of:

Anaphylactic shock: Happens due to a chronic allergic reaction (anaphylaxis).

Septic shock: Happens due to a serious bacterial infection in your bloodstream.

Neurogenic shock: Happens when your nervous system is compromised, caused by a spinal cord injury.

Drug overdoses, brain traumas, and endocrine abnormalities (such Addison's disease) are additional possible causes of distributive shock.

How Long Does Shock Last?

The duration of shock lasts is dependent on the type of shock and how quickly you get treatment. The after-effects of a shock might be severe.

When Does Shock Occur, and What Are the Symptoms?

Shock symptoms are condition - and cause-specific. One of the most typical symptoms is very low blood pressure. Some other symptoms of shock might include:

- lightheadedness, faintness, or dizziness;
- anxiety;
- confusion;
- rapid but weak heartbeat;
- shallow breathing;
- blue or gray lips and fingernails;
- fatigue;
- excessive sweating;
- pale, cool, or clammy skin;
- low or no urine.

The first step towards shock first aid therapy involves laying the patient down with their legs up.

What Is the First Aid Treatment for Shock?

The first thing you should do if you believe someone is experiencing shock is to make sure the victim is still breathing. If they are not breathing, begin rescue breathing if you are capable of doing so. If the person is breathing, check the person's breathing every five minutes until assistance arrives.

Place the individual on their back with their feet raised about 12 inches if they are awake and do not have any injuries to their head, neck, spine, or legs. Don't raise their head. If lifting their legs hurts, laying them down will help. Verify the person's comfort and warmth, and loosen any tight clothing. Provide adequate first aid and try to stop any bleeding if the patient has any visible wounds.

If they begin to drool, vomit, or bleed from their mouth, as long as they don't have a spinal injury, tilt the person's head to the side to avoid choking. If you think they may have suffered a spinal injury, do a "log roll" on the person. This involves keeping their head, neck, and back in alignment while rolling their entire body and head together.

When doing first-aid shock therapy, you should act as following:

- Give nothing to the individual to swallow, not even food or liquids
- If you think the individual might have suffered a spinal injury, don't move them
- Unless the individual is in danger, do not move them
- Don't wait for moderate symptoms of shock to get worse before getting help

What Are the Effects of Shock First Aid?

Shock has the potential to be lethal if neglected. By administering shock first aid, the person experiencing shock may be stabilized until help comes. The kind, duration, and origin of shock all affect how long it takes for treatment to begin, as well as its long-term effects.

Chapter 22: PANIC ATTACK

A panic episode can come on suddenly and intensely. Panic attack symptoms might be lessened, and their attacks can be less severe if people know what to do when they happen.

It's not uncommon for people to have panic attacks; according to one report, 13% of people will have one at some point in their lives.

Although it's impossible to tell when a panic attack will strike, having a plan for what to do in case one does happen can help one feel more in control and make managing panic attacks simpler.

This section will examine strategies for averting a panic attack as well as some all-purpose techniques for reducing anxiety. Additionally, it will examine how to help someone experiencing a panic attack.

Ways to Stop a Panic Attack

Panic episodes can bring on many psychological and physiological symptoms.

Physical manifestations may include:

- A racing heartbeat
- Sweating
- Rapid breathing

Among the emotional symptoms are:

- Sensations of anxiousness and terror
- Severe, recurring anxiety
- A sense of imminent doom

The 13 techniques that individuals can employ to help recover, control and lessen the symptoms of a panic attack are covered in the sections below.

1. Remind yourself that it will pass.

No matter how frightening it may seem at the moment, it may be helpful to keep in mind that panic attacks are temporary and won't hurt you physically.

Try to remind yourself that this is only a concentrated moment of anxiety that will pass soon.

Panic attacks usually peak in intensity within ten minutes of their onset before the symptoms start to lessen.

2. Breathe deeply

In order to calm a panic attack, deep breathing might be helpful.

Breathing might become rapid during panic episodes, and shallow breathing can result from chest constriction. Anxiety and tension might worsen with this type of breathing.

Rather, make an effort to breathe deeply and slowly, paying attention to each breath. Take deep breaths from the abdomen, filling your lungs gradually and steadily as you count to four on both your inhalation and exhalation.

Alternatively, people might practice "relaxing breath" or 4-7-8 breathing. With this method, the breath is inhaled for four seconds, held for seven, and then slowly exhaled for eight seconds.

It is important to note that deep breathing may exacerbate panic episodes in certain individuals. Instead, in these situations, the person should try concentrating on doing something they enjoy.

3. Smell some lavender

By stimulating the senses, keeping the person grounded, and providing them with something to concentrate on, a soothing scent can help reduce anxiety.

One popular traditional treatment that is well-known for inducing a feeling of peaceful relaxation is lavender. Lavender has been shown in several studies to reduce anxiety.

To smell it, try holding the oil up your nose and taking a few gentle sniffs or dabbing a little into a handkerchief. This oil is widely accessible online. However, consumers ought to limit their purchases to reliable vendors.

If the user doesn't enjoy the scent of lavender, they can try substituting it with another essential oil, such bergamot orange, lemon, or chamomile.

4. Find a peaceful spot

Anxiety attacks are frequently made worse by sights and noises. Try to locate a more tranquil area if at all feasible. This might entail stepping out of a crowded area or moving to rest against a nearby wall.

You'll be able to clear your mind and concentrate better on breathing and other coping mechanisms when you sit in a peaceful environment.

5. Focus on an object

When a person struggles with upsetting memories, emotions, or thoughts, they might feel more grounded by focusing on an object in their surroundings.

Concentrating on one stimulus can diminish other impulses. While examining the object, the individual might wish to consider its shape, who produced it, and how it feels. By using this method, the symptoms of a panic attack can be reduced.

If the person experiences panic attacks frequently, carrying a particular, well-known object might help them stay grounded. This might be a hair clip, a little toy, a seashell, or a smooth stone.

These kinds of grounding practices might be helpful for those who are coping with anxiety, trauma, and panic attacks.

6. The 5-4-3-2-1 method

A person experiencing a panic attack may feel cut off from reality. This is due to the fact that the intensity of the anxiety can overwhelm other senses.

The 5-4-3-2-1 method is a form of mindfulness and grounding approach. It assists in shifting the focus of the individual from stressful situations.

The individual using this approach should take their time and carefully go through each of the following steps:

Examine five different objects. Take a moment to consider each of these.

Look for four different sounds. Consider their origin and unique qualities.

Touch three things. Think about their temperature, texture, and intended use.

Identify two distinct scents. This might be the scent of your soap, coffee, or laundry detergent on your clothes.

Describe one taste you have. Take note of the flavor that is currently in your mouth, or taste a piece of candy.

7. Repeat a mantra

Any word, phrase, or sound that promotes power and focus can be used as a mantra. One way to help someone escape a panic episode is to recite a mantra mentally.

Something as basic as "This too shall pass" might serve as the mantra and offer comfort. It could represent something more spiritual to other people.

The individual's bodily reactions will calm down as they concentrate on softly repeating a mantra, enabling them to control their breathing and release tension in their muscles.

8. Walk or do some light exercise

A person can escape a stressful situation by walking, and the rhythm of the movement may help with breathing control.

Endorphins are chemicals released as you walk about that help to calm the body and elevate your mood. Over time, regular exercise can help lower anxiety, which may lessen the frequency or intensity of panic episodes.

9. Try muscle relaxation techniques

Tension in the muscles is another indication of panic attacks. An attack can be prevented by using muscular relaxation techniques. This is due to the possibility that other symptoms, like fast breathing, will also go away if the mind perceives that the body is relaxing.

Progressive muscular relaxation is a well-liked coping mechanism for anxiety and panic attacks.

This entails tensing and releasing certain muscles one after the other. To do this:

Tension should be held for five seconds.

As you release the muscle, say, "relax."

Allow the muscle to relax for ten seconds, then move on to the next muscle.

10. Picture your happy place

Your happy place should be where you are most relaxed. Each person will have a distinct specific location. It will be a quiet, safe, and relaxing place for them.

It might be helpful to close your eyes and visualize being in this place when an attack starts. Consider how serene that place is. Furthermore, people might picture themselves stepping barefoot on soft rugs, scorching sand, or chilly soil.

11. Take any prescribed medications

Depending on the intensity of panic attacks, medical professionals may prescribe a use-as-needed medicine. These drugs often take effect quickly.

Some contain a beta-blocker or a benzodiazepine. The beta-blocker propranolol lowers blood pressure and slows a racing heartbeat.

Xanax and Valium are two benzodiazepines that doctors frequently recommend for panic attacks.

However, people should take these medications exactly as prescribed by their doctor, as they have the potential to be quite addictive. They can have potentially fatal side effects when used with alcohol or narcotics.

Selective serotonin reuptake inhibitors are another medication that a doctor could recommend. These might help prevent panic episodes before they start.

12. Tell someone

If your attacks often happen in the same environment, such as a social space or workplace, it might be helpful to let someone know and let them know what type of assistance they can provide if it happens again.

If a panic attack occurs in public, informing another person might be helpful. They might be able to find a peaceful area and keep others from crowding in.

13. Identify your triggers

The same situations, including crowded areas, tight places, and financial difficulties, often bring on a person's panic attacks.

By learning to control or avoid their triggers, people may be able to minimize the frequency and intensity of panic episodes.

Ways to Effectively Lower Anxiety

It is beneficial for everyone to lessen the effects of anxiety. Reducing anxiety in general will also aid in the prevention of panic attacks.

The following tactics might be useful:

- Breathing exercises: It is easier to perform deep breathing during an attack if you are accustomed to using slow, deep breathing as a general relaxing technique outside of panic attacks.
- Try regular meditation: It's a terrific approach to control breathing, reduce anxiety, and foster tranquility.
- Talk to a reliable friend: Social support can reduce anxiety and provide a person with a sense of understanding and reduced sense of isolation.
- Exercise on a regular basis: This can help induce deeper sleep, release tension, and release endorphins, which uplift the mood and induce relaxation.
- Try talking therapy: If anxiety or panic is causing a person to feel anxious or panicked on a frequent basis, consider talking therapy. A mental health expert can offer guidance, assurance, and support. People in therapy can identify the sources of their anxiety and create useful coping mechanisms.
- Cognitive behavioral therapy: This kind of treatment can help patients learn coping mechanisms and become more resilient to stressful circumstances. It could be a useful strategy for treating panic episodes.

Important lifestyle adjustments can also lessen the effects of anxiety. The following strategies can help:

- minimizing or abstaining from caffeine, alcohol, and smoking;
- maintaining a nutritious diet;
- getting a restful night's sleep;
- staying hydrated.

Herbs have been used historically to treat depression and anxiety. Some of the most popular herbal medicines are accessible to purchase online, including passiflora, kava extract, and valerian.

The benefits of herbal therapies are still being studied. Consultation with a physician is usually advised prior to taking this kind of treatment.

For some people, meditation could be beneficial, but exercise might be more beneficial. Research and find the most effective strategy.

Ways to Help Someone Experiencing a Panic Attack

Some advice on how to help someone experiencing a panic attack is given in this section.

At first, try explaining a couple of the techniques mentioned above to them. Help them find a quiet place, for example, and suggest they concentrate on something close by while taking calm, deep breaths.

Introduce yourself if you don't know the person, and inquire if they need assistance. Ask about their experience with panic attacks and what methods they used to recover.

People might also try the following when someone else is experiencing a panic attack:

- Strive to keep your calm. They will feel a little more at ease as a result.

- Suggest moving to a peaceful area close by or assist them in finding one. Sitting comfortably can be really beneficial, as it enables them to concentrate on their breathing.
- Remind them that panic attacks always come to an end.
- Remain upbeat and nonjudgmental. Refrain from endorsing any unfavorable claims.
- Strike up a nice, light conversation to divert their attention and give them a sense of security.
- Refrain from advising them to calm down or that they have nothing to worry about, as this devalues their feelings.
- Stay with them. If they feel the need for solitude, make sure they stay visible.

When to Get Aid

Panic attacks can be terrifying and disorienting. A person might seek guidance and comfort from their doctor if they are concerned about having a panic attack.

Severe or recurrent panic attacks can be a symptom of panic disorder. Every year, 2-3% of Americans are afflicted by this medical condition.

A person might wish to speak with a medical expert if their panic attacks:

- Are both regular and unforeseen.
- Are interfering with day-to-day activities.
- Don't pass with home coping methods.

Medical personnel can talk a person through both long-term treatment options and short-term coping methods.

There might be similarities between the symptoms of a panic attack and a heart attack. Sweating, nervousness, and chest aches are a few of them. Someone has to get medical help right away if they think they may be having a heart attack or stroke.

While it's not always feasible to foresee when a panic attack will happen, being prepared for when one does can make the sufferer feel more in control.

Regaining control after a panic attack can be facilitated by finding a quiet place, doing deep breathing exercises, and learning grounding strategies.

Individuals can also use long-term techniques to lessen the frequency or incidence of panic episodes. These might include adopting a healthy lifestyle, attempting treatment, and learning practical techniques for managing anxiety.

Chapter 23: BREATHING DIFFICULTIES

Most individuals take breathing for granted. Breathing issues may be a recurrent occurrence for people with certain conditions. The first help for someone experiencing sudden or unforeseen breathing difficulties is covered in this section.

Breathing issues can range from:

- being short of breath;
- being unable to inhale deeply and having breathing difficulties;
- feeling like you're not breathing in enough air.

Points to Take

Having trouble breathing is frequently a medical emergency. Feeling a little exhausted after engaging in regular activity, like exercising, is an exception.

Causes

Breathing issues can have a wide range of reasons. Certain medical issues and unexpected medical emergencies are common causes.

Several medical conditions that can cause breathing issues are:

- asthma;
- low red blood cell count (Anemia);
- chronic obstructive pulmonary disease (COPD) is sometimes referred to as chronic bronchitis or emphysema;
- heart failure or heart disease;

- cancer that has spread to the lungs, or lung cancer;
- respiratory infections, such as croup, pneumonia, whooping cough, and acute bronchitis, among others;
- circumstances which limit the movement of the chest wall or diaphragm;
- certain neurological disorders.

Several health emergencies have the potential to cause breathing problems:

- heart attack;
- lung collapse (pneumothorax);
- blood clot in the lung;
- injury to the chest wall, neck, or lungs;
- high altitude pulmonary edema (hape);
- a pericardial effusion is a fluid accumulation around the heart that might prevent it from filling with blood adequately;
- pleural effusion, or potentially compressive fluid around the lungs;
- near drowning, which causes fluid to accumulate in the lungs;
- potentially fatal allergic response.

Symptoms

People who are experiencing trouble breathing frequently appear uncomfortable. They might be:

- Breathing rapidly
- Unable to breathe lying down and must sit up in order to breathe
- Extremely tensed and anxious
- Groggy or perplexed

They may also exhibit the following symptoms:

- Feeling lightheaded or dizzy

- Agony
- High temperature
- Cough
- Vomiting
- Nausea
- Pale lips, fingers, and fingernails
- Chest suddenly moving awkwardly
- Wheezing, gurgling, or making whistling sounds
- Sweating
- Difficulty speaking or Muffled voice
- Coughing up blood
- Accelerated or erratic heart rate

If an allergy is the cause of their breathing issues, they may have a rash or swelling of the face, throat, or tongue.

If the injury is making it difficult for them to breathe, the person may be bleeding or have an obvious wound.

First Aid

If someone is having trouble breathing:

- Verify the person's breathing, pulse, and airway. If necessary, start Rescue Brthing.
- Take off any tight clothing.
- Assist the patient in taking any recommended medication (e.g., an asthma inhaler or home oxygen).
- Monitor the person's breathing and heart rate. If you can no longer hear symptoms of irregular breathing, including wheezing, DO NOT assume that the patient's condition is getting better.

Any open wounds in the chest or neck need to be treated right away, especially if air bubbles start to form there. Bandage such wounds at once.

A "sucking" chest wound enables air to enter the person's chest cavity with every breath. A lung collapse may result from this. Bandage the wound using plastic wrap, a plastic bag, or petroleum jelly-covered gauze pads, sealing it on three sides and leaving one open. By doing this, a valve is created that lets trapped air exit the chest via the unsealed side while blocking air from entering the chest through the cut.

First Aid Guidelines for Treating Shortness of Breath

Shortness of breath, often known as dyspnea, has a variety of reasons, and each condition requires a distinct approach to treatment. Often, the only ways to address dyspnea is transport the patient to an emergency room or physician for assessment. In addition to diagnosing the cause of the dyspnea, medical professionals can administer extra oxygen to facilitate the sufferer's breath.

Steps for Treating Shortness of Breath

Nonetheless, there are some first-aid measures you may employ to address dyspnea, at least until an ambulance shows up or you manage to transfer the patient to a medical facility. Try these measures if you have dyspnea:

Have the victim rest. You utilize more oxygen and experience shortness of breath when you exert more energy. Imagine an amazing gym exercise. You will get dyspnea if you exercise vigorously enough. The remedy? Have a rest. I'm not sure if the sufferer is having breathing difficulties. Have a look at these symptoms of shortness of breath.

Allow the victim to lie, sit, or stand where they feel most comfortable. In order to optimize chest expansion, coaches may occasionally instruct athletes to hold their arms over their heads. The "tripod position" is a technique used by paramedics, which involves leaning forward from a chair or bed and supporting up with elbows or hands on knees. However, because each individual is unique, allow the sufferer to choose the posture that seems the most comfortable.

Use oxygen. If the sufferer has access to oxygen, this is the purpose. If the person has long-term lung issues, their physician may have warned them that breathing in too much oxygen for too long might exacerbate existing conditions. The patient should utilize oxygen during periods of dyspnea, as prescribed by a medical professional.

Address the underlying cause of dyspnea. Shortness of breath has a wide range of causes, many of which are curable. Patients with asthma, for instance, may have access to a variety of devices and medications to treat unexpected dyspnea. For treatment, lung infection victims may need to visit a physician. An ambulance may be necessary for heart attack patients.

Recall

There are several, sometimes very significant, reasons why someone may experience dyspnea. In the worst instance, breathing difficulties are brought on by a heart attack, an unexpected lung condition, or a potentially fatal poisoning.

DO NOT:

Give food or liquids to the person.

If there has been an injury to the head, neck, chest, or airways, do not move the patient unless it is essential. When moving the person, make sure their neck is protected and stabilized.

Put a cushion beneath the person's head. This can obstruct the airway.

Prior to seeking medical attention, see whether the patient's condition gets better. Get help right away.

When the situation may be more serious

In these cases the situation may be more serious and only medical support will be needed:

- Have a cold or other respiratory disease and are having breathing difficulties
- Experiencing a persistent cough for more than a few weeks
- Are coughing up blood
- Are experiencing sudden weight loss or increased perspiration during the night
- Problem sleeping or waking up at night due to difficulty in breathing
- You may find it difficult to breathe when engaging in activities you usually enjoy, such as climbing stairs
- If a kid develops a barking or wheezing cough

Prevention

In order to avoid breathing difficulties, you can:

Wear a medical alert tag and have an epinephrine pen on you if you have a history of life-threatening allergic reactions. The epinephrine pen's usage will be shown to you by your care provider.

Asthma and allergy sufferers should take steps to reduce their exposure to allergens like dust mites and mold found in the home.

DO NOT smoke, and avoid exposure to anyone who is smoking. Keep your house smoke-free at all costs.

It is imperative that you vaccinate your child against whooping cough (pertussis).

Avoid getting blood clots in your legs by getting up and moving about every few hours on a long flight. Clots, once formed, can break off and become lodged in the lungs. Raising and lowering your heels, toes, and knees while seated will help get blood pumping to your legs. Get out of the car and stretch your legs at regular intervals while you're driving.

Drop the extra pounds if you're overweight. Being overweight increases your risk of getting out of breath easily. You're also more likely to develop cardiovascular disease or have a heart attack.

If you have a history of respiratory problems, such as asthma, you should always wear a medical alert tag.

HOW TO TAKE A PULSE IN FIRST AID

One crucial first aid technique that first aiders should feel comfortable with is taking a patient's pulse. There are several justifications for why measuring a pulse is crucial, as well as various methods you might employ.

What is a pulse?

Your heart creates a pressure wave as it beats or contracts. The heart rate, which is expressed in beats per minute, can be determined by detecting and counting this pressure wave.

It is often required to compress an artery against a bone in order to feel (palpate) a pulse. Due to this, a pulse is typically only detectable at certain locations on the body.

Why is taking my pulse important?

A pulse can reveal vital information regarding the condition of a casualty. The heart rate of an individual might increase or decrease due to a variety of illnesses and medical conditions.

How do I take a pulse?

Certain places to take a pulse:

- The radial artery in the wrist
- The carotid artery in the neck
- The brachial artery in the elbow crease

You ought to compress the artery with two fingers in order to take a pulse. It may require considerable experience to locate pulses with accuracy and speed.

Once the pulse has been located, you must count to get the heart rate in beats per minute. The most precise way is to count for a full minute. Alternatively, you can count for thirty seconds and then multiply by 2.

The greatest approach to get proficient at taking a pulse is to practice! Prioritize checking your own pulse before beginning to practice on others (always with their consent!).

Chapter 24: RESPIRATORY RATE FOR ADULTS AND CHILDREN

The amount of breaths you take per minute while at rest is known as your respiratory rate. Twelve to eighteen breaths per minute is the average adult respiratory rate. Children's normal respiratory rates vary according to their age. For instance, compared to older children and teenagers, newborns and toddlers breathe more often each minute.

Normal respiratory rates often rise with activity and vary significantly depending on age.

It's crucial to understand the typical respiratory rate for your age group and how to evaluate your own because a difference in it might indicate a health issue.

The typical respiratory rates in adults and children are discussed in this section. It describes how to recognize when yours has changed and what you might be able to infer about your health from that change.

Normal Respiratory Rates In Children

Children breathe faster than adults do, and age-related variations in "normal" respiration occur. The rate ranges for youngsters are broken down as follows:

Age	Rate (Breaths Per Minute)
Newborn	30 to 60
Infant (1 to 12 months)	30 to 60
Toddler (1 to 2 years)	24 to 40

Preschooler (3 to 5 years)	22 to 34
School-aged child (6 to 12 years)	18 to 30
Adolescent (13 to 17 years)	12 to 16

Periodic Breathing In Children

Generally speaking, infants breathe far more quickly than older kids do. Furthermore, they may have periodic breathing. A child's average respiratory rate increases and decreases with periodic breathing. They could have intervals where their breathing is slower than usual, interspersed with short bursts of extremely rapid breathing.

For a parent, periodic breathing might be alarming. However, unless your kid exhibits further indications of an underlying medical illness, it's typically normal.

Normal Respiratory Rate In Adults

A person's respiratory rate should be assessed when they are at rest, not after engaging in strenuous exercise. Women generally breathe a little bit more quickly than males do.

An adult in good health breathes between 12 and 18 times each minute on average.

Periodic Breathing In Adults

Periodic variations in breathing rates in adults may indicate a medical condition. Adults who breathe in patterns of rapid, shallow breaths interspersed with intervals of sluggish or no breathing are said to have Cheyne-Stokes breathing. This kind of irregular breathing is not regarded as typical. It might be brought on by:

- Carbon monoxide poisoning
- Congestive heart failure
- Hyponatremia (Low sodium level in the blood)
- Final stages of dying
- High altitude

Elderly People

Compared to younger persons, older adults often have greater normal respiratory rates. This is particularly true for older people in long-term care institutions.

Normal Respiratory Rates During Exercise

Your muscles have to consume more oxygen to produce more energy when you exercise, which makes them work harder.

A healthy adult's resting respiratory rate typically ranges from 18 to 40 breaths per minute; with physical activity, this rate can reach 60 breaths per minute. More oxygen is able to enter your lungs due to the faster breathing.

Children who exercise also tend to breathe more quickly, and they may occasionally have moderate discomfort for a brief period.

Nonetheless, rapid breathing that is accompanied by other symptoms like coughing or wheezing is abnormal at any age and needs to be assessed by a medical practitioner.

What the Respiratory Rate Means

The rate at which your brain instructs your body to breathe may be determined by counting the breaths you take in a minute. Your body will breathe more often if the blood's oxygen content is low or if the blood's carbon dioxide content is high.

For instance, the body produces more carbon dioxide when it is severely infected. This holds even in cases where blood oxygen levels are within normal limits. To expel carbon dioxide from the body, the brain signals the body to breathe more often.

However, there are instances where this approach isn't as effective. One instance is when people take narcotic medications. These drugs lessen the brain's sensitivity to blood signaling. You could thus breathe less frequently than necessary.

Two such instances are strokes and head traumas. Both have the potential to harm the brain's respiratory center.

According to recent research, your doctor may be able to anticipate disastrous medical problems if they know your breathing rate. Research also indicates that breathing rates are not monitored as frequently as they ought to be. It has been dubbed the "ignored vital sign."

Abnormal Respiratory Rates

Both increased and decreased respiration rates may indicate a medical condition. A wide range of medical disorders can contribute to either a fast or slow rate.

Medical experts use a variety of words to describe abnormal rates, such as:
- Bradypnea is breathing that is unusually slow
- Tachypnea is an increased respiratory rate. Usually, these rapid breaths are shallow
- Dyspnea implies shortness of breath. It might happen at a regular, high, or low respiratory rate
- Hyperpnea is a prolonged, deep breathing. It may happen with or without rapid breathing
- Apnea implies literally "no breath." It is a period where breathing stops

Breathing rate and dyspnea, or shortness of breath, are two different things. The rate at which someone breathes can occasionally influence whether or not they experience dyspnea. Other times, it doesn't. Rapid breathing might make you feel out of breath. It is also possible to breathe at a modest rate without experiencing dyspnea.

Measuring Respiratory Rate

One way to calculate someone's respiratory rate is to count how many breaths they take in a minute. Since a variety of factors may influence the outcome, it's important to know how to measure accurately.

It is best to assess the rate while the subject is at rest rather than after they have moved around.

Results may change if you are aware that your breaths are being measured. It's because when individuals realize they're being observed, they frequently alter their breathing patterns. According to one study, rates were around 2.13 breaths per minute slower when the patient was aware that they were being examined.

Nurses discretely count breaths to address this issue. They count the rises and falls in your chest, frequently feigning to measure your pulse.

If you're taking a respiratory rate, keep an eye out for these other indications of a breathing issue:

Is your patient or loved one uncomfortable?

Do the neck muscles tighten up as they breathe? This is referred to as "the use of accessory muscles" to breathe in medical terminology.

Do you notice any unusual breathing noises, such as wheezing?

Does the breathing, such as the hyperventilation that can precede extreme pain or terror, appear to be a reflection of discomfort or anxiety?

Increased Respiratory Rate

A breathing rate in an adult that exceeds 20 breaths per minute is often regarded as high. A highly dangerous condition is indicated by a rate of more than 24 breaths per minute. It might not be as severe when the increased rate is attributed to a psychological disorder like a panic attack.

Respiratory rate is an important indication that cannot be overlooked. According to one study, respiratory rate is a more accurate indicator of high risk than blood pressure or heart rate.

Adults

An increased breathing rate might have a variety of reasons. Some have nothing to do with the lungs, while others do. In adults, the more typical reasons are:

Acidosis: An increase in blood acidity is accompanied by an increase in carbon dioxide levels. The respiratory rate increases as a result. Diabetes and other metabolic disorders may cause this (diabetic ketoacidosis). We call this deep, fast breathing "Kussmaul's respiration."

Asthma: Breathing rates often rise during an asthma episode. Even little increases may indicate more serious breathing issues. It's essential to monitor breathing rates closely.

Breathing too quickly can often be triggered by chronic obstructive pulmonary disease, also known as COPD. It tends to occur in those who have smoked in the past.

Dehydration: Breathing becomes more rapid when dehydrated.

Fever: When you have a fever, your body tries to cool you down by making you breathe more quickly. Breathing too quickly might indicate a condition is getting worse. When assessing a breathing rate, fever is something you should take into account.

eart problems: High breathing rates are common in people with heart failure and other cardiac disorders.

Hyperventilation: People may breathe more quickly when under stress, discomfort, rage, or panic.

Infections: Rapid breathing can be brought on by the flu, pneumonia, TB, and other illnesses.

Lung problems: The respiratory rate is often elevated by disorders including pulmonary emboli, lung cancer, or blood clots that travel to the lungs.

Overdoses: Amphetamine or aspirin overdoses can cause breathing to speed up.

Newborns

Mild conditions such as transient tachypnea of the newborn (TTN) are typical causes of a fast respiratory rate in newborns. More severe issues like respiratory distress syndrome may potentially be the reason.

Children

Fever and dehydration are the most frequent reasons for an elevated respiratory rate in children. Some claim that the breathing rate increases by five to seven breaths a minute for every degree Celsius that the body temperature raises.

That isn't always the case with kids younger than a year old. Kids who don't have a fever cannot breathe more quickly. When they do breathe more quickly, it typically increases by seven to eleven breaths per minute per degree Celsius.

Frequent causes include conditions like bronchiolitis and pneumonia. Children's breathing rates can also be accelerated by asthma and acidosis.

Decreased Respiratory Rate

A low respiratory rate, according to some experts, is less than 12 breaths per minute. Some claim that it is less than eight. Often, a low breathing rate requires attention.

While counting a child's breaths, ensure you use the rate ranges for children, and while counting an adult's breaths, use the adult ranges.

Among the reasons for lower rates are:

- Alcohol: Consuming alcohol might cause your breathing to slow down.
- Brain conditions: Breathing becomes more difficult as a result of brain damage, such as head injuries and strokes.
- Metabolic: Respiratory rate may decrease to counteract the impact of abnormal metabolic processes in the body.
- Narcotics: Whether used unlawfully or for medical reasons, certain drugs, such as narcotics, can cause breathing difficulties.
- Sleep apnea: When you have sleep apnea, your breathing can completely cease, rapidly slow down, or speed up as you sleep.

When to Contact Your Medical Professional

It is advisable to get in touch with your healthcare doctor if your breathing rate changes. This is particularly valid if you suffer from a medical condition like heart disease or asthma. Even a modest rise in breathing rate may be cause for concern.

If you work in healthcare, you should be well aware of this sometimes overlooked crucial indication. According to one study, taking a respiratory rate just before leaving the emergency department might help predict post-discharge issues.

The total amount of breaths you take in a minute is known as your respiratory rate. Generally speaking, adults breathe more slowly than kids do.

Because a number of medical disorders, some of which are significant, can alter how quickly or slowly you breathe, your respiratory rate is an essential measurement. When your breathing rate changes, it may imply that your body is not getting sufficient oxygen.

Infections, fevers, and dehydration can all cause breathing to become more rapid. Long-term medical disorders, including asthma, COPD, and heart issues, can also cause this. Drugs, alcohol, sleep apnea, brain traumas, and metabolic problems can slow down breathing.

Speak with a medical expert if you see any changes in your breathing rate. You may have a medical issue that requires attention.

When it comes to your health, your blood pressure and pulse might be the first metrics that spring to mind. However, breathing rate is equally, if not more, significant. Variations in breathing patterns can indicate breathing abnormalities.

Understanding the variations in typical respiratory rates between adults and children is crucial. Knowing a child's breathing range will help you identify whether a kid is breathing too quickly or too slowly.

Chapter 25: THE ULTIMATE PREPPER FIRST AID KIT

These days, almost everyone carries a little first aid bag or kit with them. A first aid kit is now essential, whether it is kept in the trunk of your car, at home, or work. It truly isn't difficult to understand why. Everyone wants to be ready, just in case something goes wrong. It is best to have a basic first-aid kit on hand for emergencies.

What about a first aid pack designed for preppers that can handle most or all emergency scenarios?

The following is how to achieve that in this comprehensive first-aid guide.

How to Prep Yourself Medically

Before we discuss what should be in your DIY first aid kit, make sure you're prepared medically. Acquiring the necessary resources is one thing; understanding how to use them is quite another.

Furthermore, we won't lie. Confidence in one's medical knowledge feels good. So get medically prepping!

Learn life-saving skills

It is necessary to acquire life-saving skills if you wish to be ready for SHTF. This is a list of skills you should acquire:

CPR or cardiopulmonary resuscitation

While it's quite simple, doing CPR on someone may actually save their life. You can take a lot of courses to earn a certification proving that you are capable of doing CPR on people.

Heimlich Maneuver

Numerous accounts exist of strangers doing the Heimlich Maneuver on someone who is about to choke on something. That's the reason why learning it is beneficial.

We advise you to become proficient in both the adult and infant/child Heimlich Maneuver. If the adult movement is used improperly on a child, it can cause more harm than good; therefore, training is essential.

Using an Automated External Defibrillator (AED)

These days, you may find this technology anywhere—in malls, companies, and schools. When a patient has sudden cardiac arrest, an AED is a portable medical device that evaluates the patient's heart rhythm and decides whether a shock is necessary. To use an AED, you do need to have received the appropriate training to get certified.

Read Up On Medical Procedures

You are not required to read the same books that doctors and medical students do. However, it might be useful to have a rudimentary awareness of simple operations like stitching wounds. At least, if you ever have to undergo medical treatment, you won't be completely lost. In light of this, we advise you to keep a first aid manual in your prepper first aid box.

Acquaint Yourself With Meds

Purchasing several medications and cramming them into your homemade first aid kit is pointless if you don't know which ones are for what. Russian Roulette medical version, anyone? Taking medication intended to treat allergies or stomach problems is the last thing you should do.

Which Medications Are Essential To Have In Your Prepper First Aid Kit

Proper medication supply is one thing you want to have on hand for long-term survival. You can save lives by stockpiling medications or, at the very least, understanding what to buy.

The following items are suggested for your homemade first-aid kit:

Inflammation and Pain Meds

Ibuprofen (Advil): for those pesky back and knee issues, having some ibuprofen in your prepper first aid box will be quite beneficial. Inflammation can be a real pain in the ass, and nobody likes to deal with it when running is muscular soreness.

Naproxen (Aleve): women who have uncomfortable cramps during their periods often find relief using Naproxen.

Acetylsalicylic Acid (Aspirin): fever and pain that are worsened by other conditions are treated with ASA. Along with being a fantastic overall pain reliever, it also partially functions as a blood thinner, which is beneficial for avoiding blood clots and strokes. Conversely, those who suffer from bleeding issues (hemophilia) have to exercise caution about consuming certain foods.

Acetaminophen (Tylenol): this can be used to treat mild to moderate headache and toothache discomfort. Great for fevers as well. Stock up on it for your prepared first aid pack, as it will help you become more resilient to pain.

Gastro Meds

Calcium Carbonate (Tums Regular Strength): heartburns are the worst, and so are acid indigestion and stomach upset. Use calcium carbonate as an antacid to relieve the pain as soon as possible.

Bismuth Subsalicylate (Pepto-Bismol): this medication, often referred to as pink bismuth, is used to treat indigestion, diarrhea, gas, and stomach aches.

Loperamide Hydrochloride (Imodium): the last thing you want is traveler's diarrhea; therefore, it's smart to include this in your homemade first aid kit as a backup.

Topical Meds

Antiseptics (Dettol Antiseptic Liquid, Betadine, and Neosporin): one of the things you should be concerned about if you have an open wound is getting a terrible infection. Keeping antiseptics on hand is, therefore, essential. It effectively reduces the risk of infection and sepsis when used for general wound cleansing.

Burn Gel

Burn gel is an effective treatment that can help control and reduce the pain associated with first-degree burns.

Hydrocortisone Cream

This cream is frequently used to treat a variety of skin issues, including rashes, allergies, and insect bites. It will lessen the swelling as well as the irritation.

Anti-Fungal

The medication is a fungicide that cures ringworms, thrush, athlete's foot, and other conditions. It may be a lifesaver in the outdoors and a useful addition to your prepper first aid pack.

Topical Analgesics and Decongestants

Simply put, Vicks. Apply some Vicks to relieve coughs and other symptoms, and you should be set to go.

Specialized Meds

Insulin: since diabetes is actually rather widespread, whether you have the disease or know someone who does, stock up on this medication immediately. It is recommended to discuss long-term insulin preparation and stockpiling with your medical provider.

Beta Agonists (Ventolin): asthma is quite fatal. When SHTF, you want to be ready because, as asthmatics, you know how unexpected it can be.

Antihistamines (Claritin): antihistamines are ideal for controlling your allergies and dealing with them so that you don't have allergic reactions that lead you to lose consciousness or, worse, go wild and scratch them.

Epinephrine Pen: when acute allergies strike, breathing becomes easier with an EpiPen shot. An epipen is often used in an emergency.

Phenylephrine (Sudafed PE; 4-Way Nasal Spray): while you might not think much of nasal or sinus congestion, it hurts when it hits. You get headaches, stuffy noses, and facial congestion. You'll feel as though your face and head are both heavy. Phenylephrine is the most efficient way to deal with it.

Ammonia Inhalant (Dynarex Ammonia): smelling ammonia inhalant, often known as smelling salts, is a terrific approach to jolt someone back to consciousness after they've lost consciousness or feel dizzy.

Oral Rehydration Salts (Equalyte; Pedialyte): after treating diarrhea, you should take oral rehydration salts to aid in electrolyte replenishment.

Antibiotics (Amoxicillin): though antibiotic implies "against life," it's almost a lifeline when you have an unpleasant injury that is prone to infection. Antibiotics prevent diseases by eliminating germs, thereby saving your life.

Miscellaneous

Soap: nothing keeps you cleaner than a simple soap and water routine, especially when it comes to bandaging wounds. In addition to being quite affordable, soap hurts far less than other chemicals for cleansing wounds. It's an essential component of every do-it-yourself first aid kit.

Sunscreen: ever spent time in the sun and gotten a nasty sunburn? Well, if you intend to spend a lot of time outside, it pays to use sunscreen. In addition to shielding you from sunburn, it also keeps skin cancer at bay. Those, in our opinion, are sufficient justifications for stockpiling sunscreen.

Bug Spray: a simple insect or mosquito bite can cause some quite bothersome sores or consequences. While busy trying to survive, you don't want to worry about bugs. Use bug spray.

Situation Specific Kits: it's fine to have one survivalist first aid kit, but what about having many kits for different scenarios? We are aware that you are shaking in your boots. Being organized and ahead of things is the essence of prepping.

With these scenario-specific kits you may have on hand, we're bringing the preparation of your DIY first aid kit to the next level:

Wounds & General Trauma

Alcohol: the first thing to do is to consider purchasing some strong booze. Not a whiskey bottle, please. Authentic medical alcohol for disinfecting.

Gauze: you need the right tools to complete the job effectively, and gauze is a must-have item for any homemade first-aid kit. It helps in post-surgical wound and deep wound healing.

Gauze Bandages: we love gauze bandages for a few great reasons. They help in the quicker healing of wounds due to their superior ventilation. Secondly, they absorb excess moisture from the area around wounds. The secret to having an injury heal more rapidly is to keep it dry!

Gauze Clips: gauze clips are needed to hold gauze bandages in place if you have any. Moreover, you can reuse them, provided you keep them in excellent shape.

First Aid Bandages and Plasters

These will work perfectly for cuts, scratches, and general wounds, preventing the severity of your injury. You'll be set to go once you slap them on.

Hydrogen Peroxide

You can purchase any other antiseptic for your first aid kit, but is it also suitable for use as a mouthwash? So using hydrogen peroxide as a mouthwash is safe. Simply combine two parts water and one part hydrogen peroxide, and you're set to go.

Hemostatic Agents (Celox; QuikClot; Hemcon)

Hemostatic drugs are easily obtained and are often used in the military due to their exceptional ability to stop severe bleeding on the battlefield. If they are using it for serious trauma situations on the battlefield, then you need these in your survivalist first aid kit.

Triangular Bandages

This kind of bandage is triangular in design and is quite adaptable. Asides from being a tourniquet, it can be used as a sling.

Chest Seals

A sucking chest wound is any puncture wound, including gunshots and stab wounds. These kinds of wounds carry a significant risk of lung collapse. It goes without saying that you cannot DIY this thus having a chest seal on hand is essential as these kinds of wounds are the only applications for chest seals.

Surgical Tapes

Use surgical tape to hold your bandages and wound dressings in place. Another option is Durapore tape, a high-strength adhesive tape with several applications. Large dressings can be fastened together with it.

Eye Irrigating Solution

These eyewashes, which come in bottles, contain a sterile solution that you can use to wipe your eyes. This is the cure for those times when you have an itchy eye, or something gets trapped in your eye, and you simply can't seem to get it out. Quite helpful when there isn't access to clean water to wash your eyes out.

Trauma Shears

Trauma shears, which paramedics and EMTs mostly use, allow you to cut off garments during emergencies without inadvertently stabbing the injured. It's made to swiftly and safely cut off clothing.

CPR Mask

We hope you are certified in CPR because, if so, a CPR mask will make the process go more smoothly for you. If you have a CPR mask handy, you can do rescue breathing without risk.

Diagnostic Kit

Thermometers: quite simple to obtain, you can purchase a conventional or digital thermometer. To be safe, we advise adding both to your prepper first aid pack. Possessing both at your disposal is a brilliant idea.

Blood Pressure Monitor: if high blood pressure is not controlled, it can be harmful and cause several health issues, including heart disease.

To stay on top of things, you might wish to get a blood pressure monitor. Similar to the thermometer, you have two options for measuring blood pressure: a sphygmomanometer, which is a classic type of monitor, or an electronic one that does all the work for you.

Stethoscopes: stethoscopes are a well-known tool used by doctors to listen to sounds that the body makes. It is possible to listen to a person's respiration, pulse, and even the condition of their intestines.

Naturally, none of that will matter if you are unable to understand what you are hearing. In order to maximize the use of your stethoscope, it is important to possess pertinent expertise in that area.

Otoscopes: this is a tool that allows you to see inside the ears. You can view the eardrum and the ear canal with this.

While you might not give your ears much thought, when something goes wrong, things can go rather bad very quickly. For instance, how easily you can lose your sense of balance.

Fracture Kit

Splint: a splint is used to keep a fracture in place, which can occur anywhere and at any time. We advise adding a SAM splint to your homemade first aid package. This versatile splint has shown to be quite helpful in a variety of circumstances.

Orthopedic Cast: you've got your splint. You now require a cast. What distinguishes the two? A cast extends all the way around, but a splint doesn't. For certain fractures, a complete wrap-around is necessary to maintain alignment. An orthopedic cast is thus necessary.

Cast Liner/Undercast Padding: an improper liner might cause skin irritation from a splint or cast. It is essential to place padding around the fracture to offer protection and comfort.

Oral and Dental Kit

Oral Analgesic Gel: oral analgesic gels are a dental pain reliever that acts as a local anesthetic. The painful area of your mouth is numbed by it. Dental pain is horrible, but oral analgesic gels are a blessing.

Extraction Forceps: in the worst situation, when you have no choice, extraction forceps may be necessary in an emergency dental situation. Having forceps is going to be a better choice than a set of rusty pliers going into your mouth.

Cheek Retractors: we wouldn't really want to undertake any dental work at all if given the option, but occasionally, circumstances force us to take on do-it-yourself dental treatment. Cheeks retractors are useful in this situation. Cheek retractors help keep the lips wide and provide a clear view of those brilliant whites.

Dental Mirrors: have you ever tried using a flashlight and a mirror to examine the back of your mouth? It isn't possible, though. Believe us when we say so. On the other hand, dental mirrors make it quite simple to examine your teeth and check for cavities.

Temporary Dental Cement: temporary dental cement is your friend when you can't get to the dentist quickly enough. MacGyver-ing your tooth? Ignore it. Grab a kit. Finding them is not too difficult, and utilizing them is not complicated.

Surgical Kit

Scalpels and Dissection Kit: lay down that machete. It is not advisable to use a blade so large to remove a comparatively little splinter. Have some of the necessary instruments on hand if you want to do a surgical procedure anywhere other than an operating room.

When in doubt, the safest course of action to ensure proper healing is to stitch up the wound.

Additionally, the most self-explanatory items you'll need for your prepper first aid kit are:

- Hot and cold packs
- Towels
- Headlamp
- Reusable surgical gowns
- Medical nitrile gloves
- Surgical masks
- Cotton swabs
- Needles and syringes
- Sterile cotton balls

Birth Kit

Childbirth is still possible with the TEOTWAWKI; thus, it's important to prepare a birth kit in case you need it. You should not attempt to do this on your own, particularly if you have a newborn in the house.

IV Kit

IV kits come extremely handy for administering medication, fluid replacement, and performing blood transfusions, should the need arise. This is another thing you cannot do yourself, and we also wouldn't want you to try.

While the amount of information on medical supplies for preppers may seem daunting, we would much rather be overloaded than left unimpressed.

Naturally, you don't need to get every item on our above list. While it's only intended to be a reference, you can always add your own preferred goods or brands to make your DIY first aid kit uniquely yours.

CONCLUSION

Everyone will either receive or administer first aid at some time in their lives. Prompt action can raise the chances that an emergency will end well. It is crucial to provide as much help as you can provide the victim, but the greatest result for any victim can be guaranteed if the appropriate medical specialists in your community are notified as soon as possible. Always make sure the area is safe before helping a victim.

While waiting for emergency assistance, victims of various medical problems need to know how to do CPR and first aid to improve their chances of survival. For this reason, everyone need to sign up for the easily accessible online certification programs.

Training in CPR and First Aid equips the practitioner with the fundamental knowledge and abilities to handle a variety of medical situations, as well as the self-assurance needed to administer medical care. All individuals are welcome to participate in the programs, regardless of age or educational background, as there are no minimum requirements.

When administering first aid, it's critical to keep oneself safe from infectious diseases and other dangers. To help protect yourself:

It is advisable to always look out for potential threats to your safety before approaching someone who is ill or injured.

• Keep your hands away from vomit, blood, and other body fluids.

• Put on safety gear, such as vinyl or nitrile gloves, while administering care to someone who has an open wound or when executing rescue breathing.

• As soon as you finish administering first aid, wash your hands with soap and water.

Many times, administering simple first aid can prevent a minor problem from getting worse. First aid in a medical emergency might potentially save a life. If someone have a significant illness or injury, they should get follow-up treatment from a medical expert.

Now we have also finally come to the bonuses I have decided to give you with this book to increase your emergency preparedness.

BONUS #1

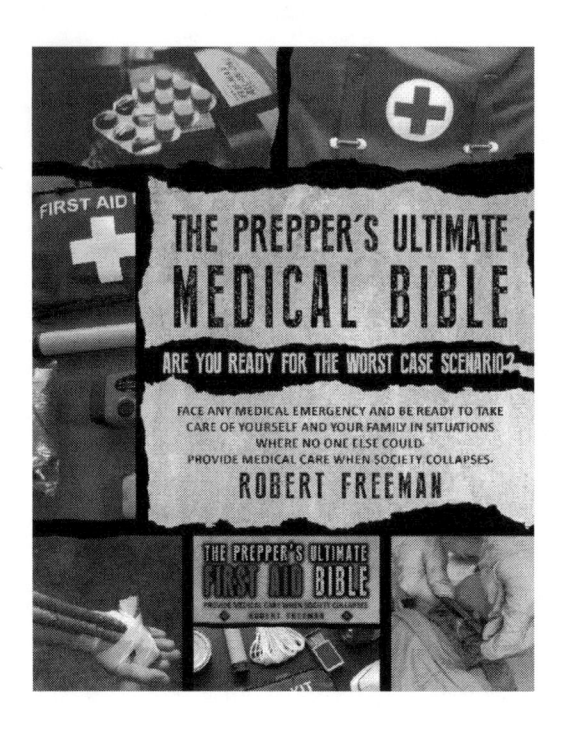

Enhance your medical training with the first bonus: THE PREPPER'S ULTIMATE MEDICAL BIBLE book in a downloadable and printable PDF version:

Scan this code and get your free printable PDF file

BONUS #2

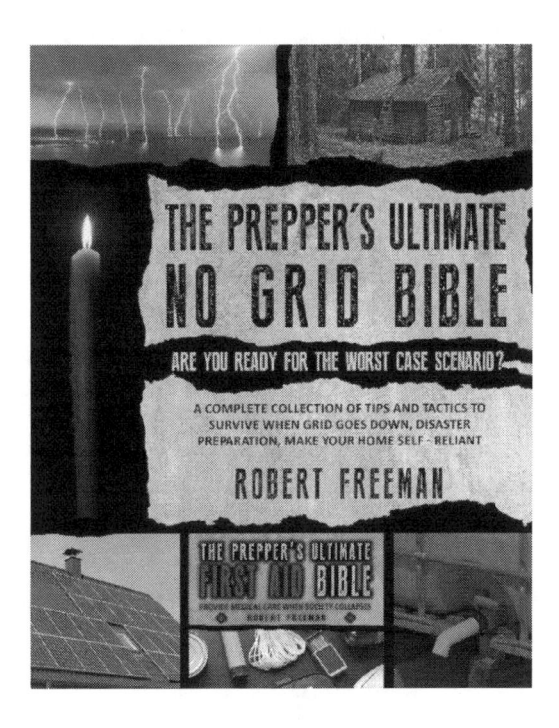

Enhance your preparedness with the second bonus: THE PREPPER'S ULTIMATE NO GRID BIBLE book in a downloadable and printable PDF version:

Scan this code and get your free printable PDF file

BONUS #3

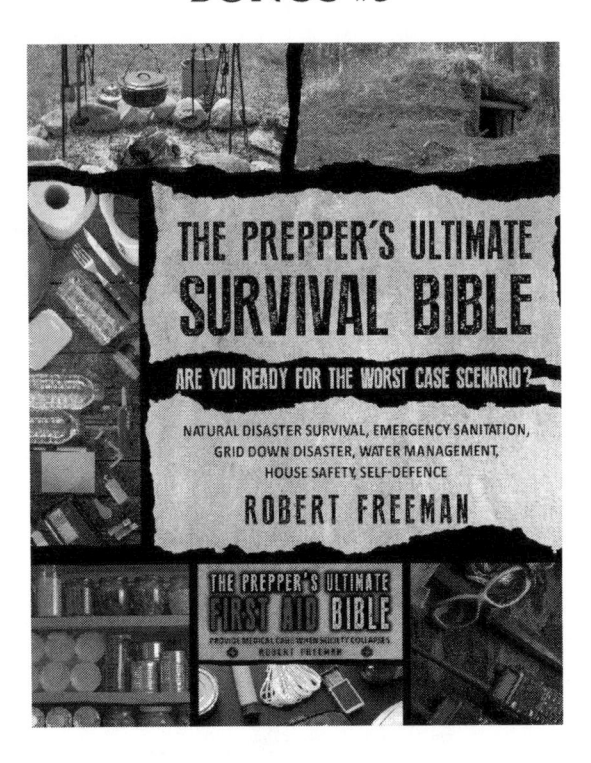

Enhance your preparedness with the third bonus: THE PREPPER'S ULTIMATE SURVIVAL BIBLE book in a downloadable and printable PDF version:

Scan this code and get your free
printable PDF file

Made in the USA
Middletown, DE
04 January 2025